Dept. of Haem
Whipps Cross Hospital

LONDON  E11-1NR

# BONE
# MARROW
# BIOPSIES
# REVISITED

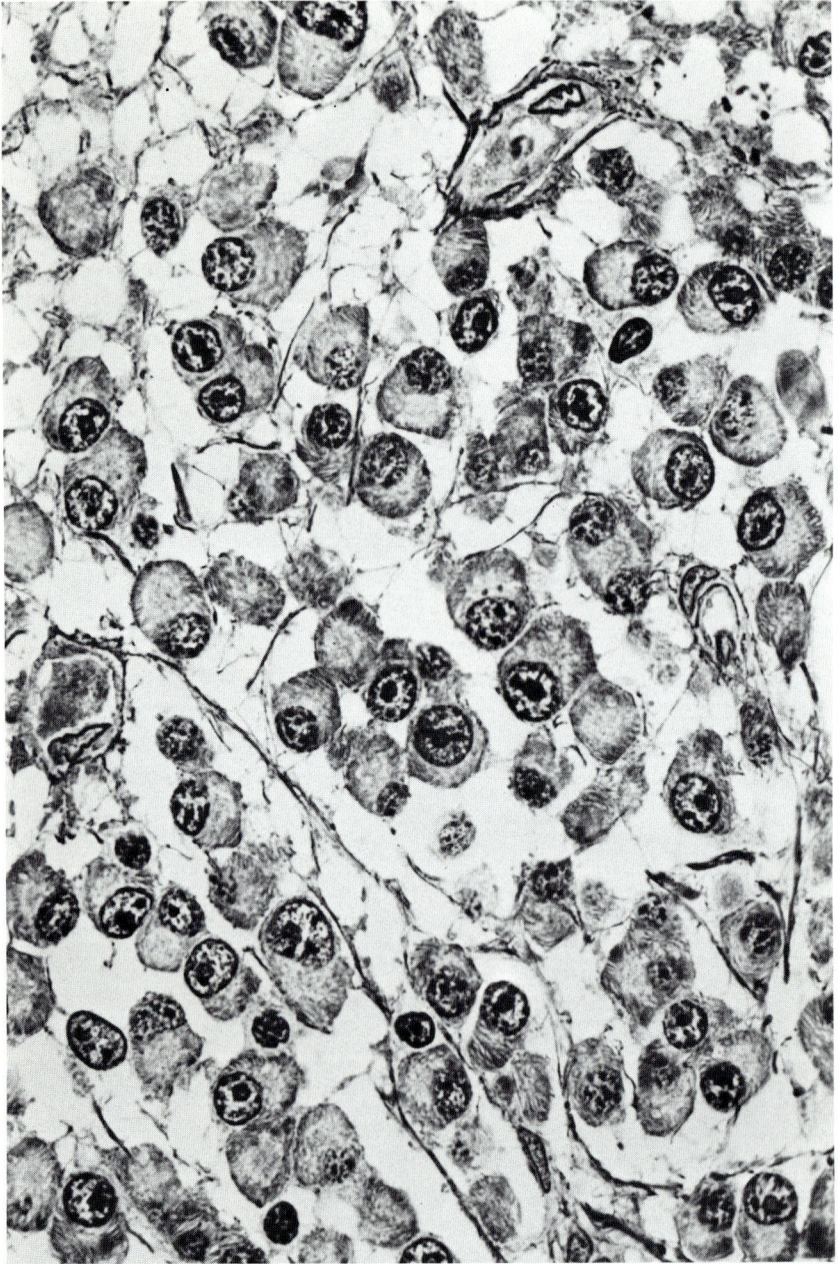

Multiple myeloma, plasmacytic type. Gomori. × 600.

R. Bartl
B. Frisch
R. Burkhardt

# BONE MARROW BIOPSIES REVISITED

## A New Dimension for Haematologic Malignancies

2nd, revised edition
78 figures, 18 tables, 16 colour plates, 1985

**KARGER**

S. Karger · Basel · München · Paris · London · New York · Tokyo · Sydney

**Reiner Bartl**

Prof. Dr. med., Abteilung für Knochenmarksdiagnostik,
Medizinische Klinik Innenstadt der Universität München
(Director: Prof. Dr. E. Buchborn), München (FRG),
and Abteilung für Hämatomorphologie, Institut für Hämatologie,
Gesellschaft für Strahlen- und Umweltforschung mbH, München (FRG)

**Bertha Frisch**

Prof., MD, Institute of Hematology,
Tel-Aviv Municipal Governmental Medical Center, and
The Sackler School of Medicine, Tel-Aviv University, Tel Aviv (Israel)

**Rolf Burkhardt**

Prof. Dr. med., Head of the Abteilung für Knochenmarksdiagnostik,
Medizinische Klinik Innenstadt der Universität München
(Director: Prof. Dr. E. Buchborn), München (FRG),
and of the Abteilung für Hämatomorphologie, Institut für Hämatologie,
Gesellschaft für Strahlen- und Umweltforschung mbH, München (FRG)

1st edition 1982
German translation: Karger, 1984

National Library of Medicine, Cataloging in Publication
  Bartl, R. (Reiner)
  Bone marrow biopsies revisited: a new dimension for haematologic malignancies
  R. Bartl, B. Frisch, R. Burkhardt. – Basel, New York: Karger, 1985.
  Includes bibliographies and index.
  1. Biopsy, Needle   2. Bone Marrow Examination   3. Hematologic Disease – diagnosis
  4. Neoplasms – diagnosis   I. Frisch, B. (Bertha)   II. Burkhardt, R. (Rolf)   III. Title
  WH 380 B289b
  ISBN 3–8055–3937–1

# Contents

Contents

# Colour Plates

# Foreword

In the past 40 years bone marrow aspiration cytology has been the basis of morphological investigation and diagnosis. Well-made, well-fixed, and well-stained preparations from easily aspirated samples provide much information on the structure of the marrow fragments, on the overall cellularity of the marrow, on the relative proportions of the cells in the different haemopoietic cell lineages. Above all they provide exquisite cytomorphological detail and permit the recognition of abnormal haemopoietic cells and of cells not normally present in the marrow. Material yielding information of such quality cannot be replaced, and will continue to be the basis of morphological diagnosis. However, its very success has led to a long-standing neglect, now happily no longer relevant, of other methods. Even in the best aspiration preparations the spatial distribution of the haemopoietic cells and the anatomic relation between the cells and the vascular, fatty, and bony structures can never be seen. Successful methods for preparing histological sections of aspirated fragments go some way to remedy the deficiency, but they also emphasize the fact that aspirated fragments are selected samples because the suction required to dislodge them inevitably tears them away from the bony trabeculae.

Because the distribution of haemopoietic cells is not the same in the intertrabecular regions, which make up the bulk of aspiration samples, and in the paratrabecular regions, even the best aspiration samples may not reflect faithfully the distribution of the cells in the marrow. This deficiency of marrow aspiration has been accepted, or ignored, and was not even recognized until a proper study of trephine biopsy sections, as described in this volume, was made.

More serious problems arise when marrow is aspirated with difficulty, when the fragments tend to clot and do not spread well, when marrow juice but no fragments can be obtained, when only blood is obtained, or when nothing at all can be aspirated even with strong suction or after attempts at several different sites. Until fairly recently, the technique of trephine biopsy

was reserved for these cases. The procedure was done relatively infrequent-
ly, a variety of trephine needles of different sizes were used, and the bony
cores required decalcification before sectioning. In all too many cases the
resulting sections were of poor quality, with gross crushing artifacts, and
poorly preserved cytological detail in the few areas where the architecture
was better preserved.

For many years a few far-sighted individuals, among them *Matthew
Block* and *Rolf Burkhardt,* have insisted on the inadequacy of aspiration in
the morphological assessment of the bone marrow, and they have empha-
sized the great importance of high quality trephine sections as primary
material and not merely as supplements to aspiration preparations. Accep-
tance of their contention, slow in coming, was partly dependent on the
realization that aspiration was a poor method of establishing marrow
involvement in Hodgkin's disease, other lymphomas and malignant diseases. As it came to be recognized that different methods of treatment were
required at different stages, staging procedures became part of the obliga-
tory work-up before appropriate treatment could be planned and as a result,
bone marrow trephine biopsy has come to be used far more frequently in
the past decade. However, the quality of many preparations is often, frank-
ly, unsatisfactory.

Professor *Burkhardt* and his colleagues have, over the years, perfected
their techniques for preparing semi-thin undecalcified plastic-embedded
sections of bone marrow cores, and for staining them to reveal cytological
features in astonishing detail. Examination of his preparations opens a new
world to the observer. After becoming familiar with these superb preparations, one becomes reluctant to look at conventional decalcified paraffin
embedded sections. A few years ago, one of my colleagues had the privilege
of learning the techniques for preparing semi-thin undecalcified plastic
embedded sections in Professor *Burkhardt's* department and we have come
to rely heavily on them. The technique can be adapted, as described in this
volume, for applying cytochemical reactions, and in fresh-frozen material
for the immunological identification of specific cell constituents.

The routine use of high quality trephine sections makes it possible to
open up many fields of enquiry which simply could not be carried out at all
on aspiration samples, or on inferior section material. This book brings
together the results of systematic studies on the use of trephine sections over
a 10-year period in over 2,000 cases of haematological malignant disease
and illustrates the enormous scope the technique provides in haemato-
oncological enquiry.

In particular, these authors have shown that quantitative studies can be made on the sections and in consequence they can contribute to the assessment of marrow function in health and disease. It is to be hoped that the technique will now become part of the expertise in haematological practice everywhere.

*D.A.G. Galton*
MA, MD, FRCP, Professor of Haematological Oncology,
Honorary Director, MRC Leukaemia Unit,
Consultant Physician, Hammersmith Hospital, London, England

# Acknowledgments

The authors would like to express their gratitude to all colleagues who referred patients or sent biopsies, to the technical staff of the laboratory, especially to Mrs. *B. Buchenrieder,* Mrs. *W. Sommerfeld* and Mrs. *H. Muthmann* for the histologic preparation, to Dr. *K. Jäger,* Dr. *G. Kettner* and Dr. *G. Mahl* for their cooperation in evaluating and computerizing the material, to Mrs. *I. Weltmeier,* Mrs. *G. Huber,* Mrs. *G. Stark,* Mrs. *I. Pascher,* Mrs. *F. Haag,* Mrs. *H. Petry,* Mrs. *I. Werner* and Mrs. *I. Wiktorin* for typing and illustrating the manuscript, and, last but not least, to the publisher Dr. *T. Karger* and his editorial and technical staff. This work was supported by the Medical Faculty of the University of Munich, the Gesellschaft für Strahlen- und Umweltforschung mbH, Neuherberg/Munich, the Deutsche Forschungsgemeinschaft, Bonn, and Carl Zeiss, Oberkochen.

# 1   Introduction

It is generally accepted in medical practice that the diagnosis of a malignancy must be established by histology before treatment is instituted [10, 16]. Nevertheless this has not been, and still is not the case in haematologic oncology, in which a bone marrow biopsy is only required when smears of the aspirate did not provide the diagnosis, or a dry tap was obtained [11]. Consequently the early stages of myelofibrosis for long went unrecognized as they cannot be revealed by aspiration [2, 4]. Likewise the evaluation of leukaemic and non-leukaemic lymphatic proliferations in the bone marrow was greatly limited as long as their investigation was confined to cytologic methods. More recently, the inclusion of bone marrow biopsy in the assessment of malignant lymphomas has contributed to the early diagnosis and more effective treatment of these disorders [5, 12, 14]. Moreover bone marrow structure itself may be informative independent of cytology. Cells of the haematopoietic system, both normal and malignant, are distinguished by their motility and their proliferative capacity even outside their usual confines, and the bone marrow which produces them does not consist only of their precursors.

The blood-forming elements are subject to a complicated structural organization within the bone marrow, indicating the formative influence of this organ [2, 8, 18]. Following damage to the bone marrow or after its transplantation to another site, haematopoiesis is only initiated after reconstruction of the stroma [17]. Particular regions of the bone marrow have specific effects on the differentiation of the blood cells: the 'haematopoietic inductive microenvironment' [1, 8, 15]. Once these facts are recognized and, in addition, the leukaemias themselves show various growth and distribution patterns within the bone marrow, it is clear that the participation of various forms of tissue organization will have to be taken into consideration in the development of haematopoietic malignancies and in their response to therapy.

The increasing use of bone marrow biopsies was promoted by the introduction of improved instruments for taking them and of better techniques for their histologic preparation [2, 3, 6, 7, 9, 13]. However, before the introduction of bone marrow biopsy as a routine procedure into clinical practice, the indications must be clearly defined, and, in particular, whether a bone biopsy should be regarded as complementary or as an alternative to aspiration cytology.

The contents of this book are the results of the first systematic attempt to derive diagnostic and prognostic information from bone marrow histology in a large series of patients with haematologic malignancies. Each chapter on one of the main disease groups comprises a survey of the literature, a compilation of our recent observations (to some extent already published in the journals listed in the references) and the consequent implications for medical practice.

## References

1   Boggs, D.R.: The hematopoietic microenvironment. New Engl. J. Med. *302:* 1359–1360 (1980).
2   Burkhardt, R.: Farbatlas der klinischen Histopathologie von Knochenmark und Knochen (Springer, Berlin 1970).
3   Burkhardt, R.: Bone marrow histology; in Catovsky, Methods in hematology. The leukemic cell, pp. 49–86 (Churchill Livingstone, Edinburgh 1981).
4   Burkhardt, R.; Bartl, R.; Beil, E.; Demmler, K.; Hoffmann, E.; Kronseder, A.; Langegger, H.; Saar, U.; Ulrich, M.; Wiemann, H.: Myelofibrosis-osteosclerosis syndrome. Review of literature and histomorphology; in Advances in the biosciences, vol. 16, pp. 9–56 (Pergamon Press, Oxford/Vieweg, Braunschweig 1975).
5   Come, S.E.; Chabner, B.A.: Staging in non-Hodgkin's lymphoma: approach, results and relationship to histopathology; in Canellos, Clinics in haematology, vol. 8, pp. 645–656 (Saunders, Philadelphia 1979).
6   Frisch, B.; Bartl, R.; Burkhardt, R.: Bone marrow biopsy in clinical medicine: an overview. Haematologia *3:* 245–285 (1982).
7   Jamshidi, K.; Swaim, W.R.: Bone marrow biopsy with unaltered architecture: a new biopsy device. J. Lab. clin. Med. *77:* 335–342 (1971).
8   Knospe, W.H.: Hematopoietic microenvironment: role of sinusoidal microcirculation and other stromal elements, in Aplastic anemia, pp. 95–107 (Japan Medical Research Foundation, University of Tokyo Press, Tokyo 1978).
9   Krause, J.R.: Bone marrow biopsy (Churchill Livingstone, New York 1981).
10  Myers, W.P.: Cancer and internal medicine; an internist's approach to cancer and its medical manifestations; in Beeson, McDermott, Wyngaarden, Textbook of medicine, pp. 1898–1906 (Saunders, Philadelphia 1979).
11  Rappaport, H.: Histologic criteria for diagnosis and classification of acute leukemias; in Mathé, Pouillart, Schwarzenberg, Nomenclature, methodology and results of clinical trials in acute leukemias, pp. 35–42 (Springer, Berlin 1973).

12  Rosenberg, S.A.: Current concepts in cancer. Non-Hodgkin's lymphoma: selection of treatment on the basis of histologic type. New Engl. J. Med. *301:* 924–928 (1979).

13  Rowden, G.; Sacher, R.A.; More, N.S.: Plastic embedded specimens for evaluation of bone marrow; in Roath, Topical reviews in haematology, vol. II, pp. 1–92 (Wright, Bristol 1982).

14  Sutcliffe, S.B.J.; Timothy, A.R.; Lister, T.A.: Staging in Hodgkin's disease; in Canellos, Clinics in haematology, vol. 8, pp. 593–609 (Saunders, Philadelphia 1979).

15  Trentin, J.J.: Influence of hematopoietic organ stroma (hematopoietic inductive microenvironment) on stem cell differentiation; in Gordon, Regulation of hematopoiesis, vol. 1, pp. 161–186 (Appleton-Century-Crofts, New York 1970).

16  Ultmann, J.F.; Golomb, H.M.: Principles of neoplasia: approach to diagnosis and management; in Isselbacher, Adams, Braunwald, Petersdorf, Wilson, Harrison's principles of internal medicine; 9th ed., pp. 1583–1597 (McGraw-Hill, New York 1980).

17  Umehara, S.: Bone marrow stroma in aplastic anemia; in Aplastic anemia, pp. 109–121 (Japan Medical Research Foundation, University of Tokyo Press, Tokyo 1978).

18  Weiss, L.; Chen, L.T.: The organization of hematopoietic cords and vascular sinuses in bone marrow. Blood Cells *1:* 617–638 (1975).

# 2  Patients and Methods

## Patients

In this retrospective study, a total of 2,225 patients with haematologic malignancies was investigated since 1970; the follow-up period ranged from 1 to 10 years. Bone marrow biopsy was performed in 2,055 of these patients as part of the initial investigation, the remaining 170 had already received specific therapy and the biopsies were taken for monitoring. In 410 cases sequential biopsies (up to 8 biopsies in 1 patient) were available to assess the course of the disease. The distribution in the major disease groups with bone marrow manifestations was as follows: chronic myeloproliferative disorders (MPD) 400, adult acute leukaemias (AL) 182, multiple myeloma (MM) 220, non-Hodgkin's lymphomas (NHL) 465, and Hodgkin's disease (HD) 93. Furthermore, 568 HD patients with negative biopsies were included to assess the prognostic value of non-specific bone marrow reactions. 158 biopsies of healthy individuals were evaluated for comparison. Informed consent was obtained in all cases.

## Biopsy Techniques and Histologic Preparations

3,000 bone marrow biopsies were taken from the anterior and posterior iliac crests. The myelotomy drill was used in 85% and the Jamshidi needle in 15% of the cases. The former provided biopsy cores with a mean size of 4 $\times$ 18 mm (accepted minimal size 4 $\times$ 8 mm), the latter had mean dimensions of 2 $\times$ 15 mm (accepted minimal size 2 $\times$ 10 mm) (fig. 1, 2). Both were employed for histomorphometric measurements. The cores obtained by myelotomy may be halved longitudinally and one half used for plastic embedding and the other for imprints, histochemistry and electron microscopy (fig. 3, 4). All biopsies were fixed, dehydrated and embedded in methylmethacrylate without decalcification, and semi-thin sections were cut at

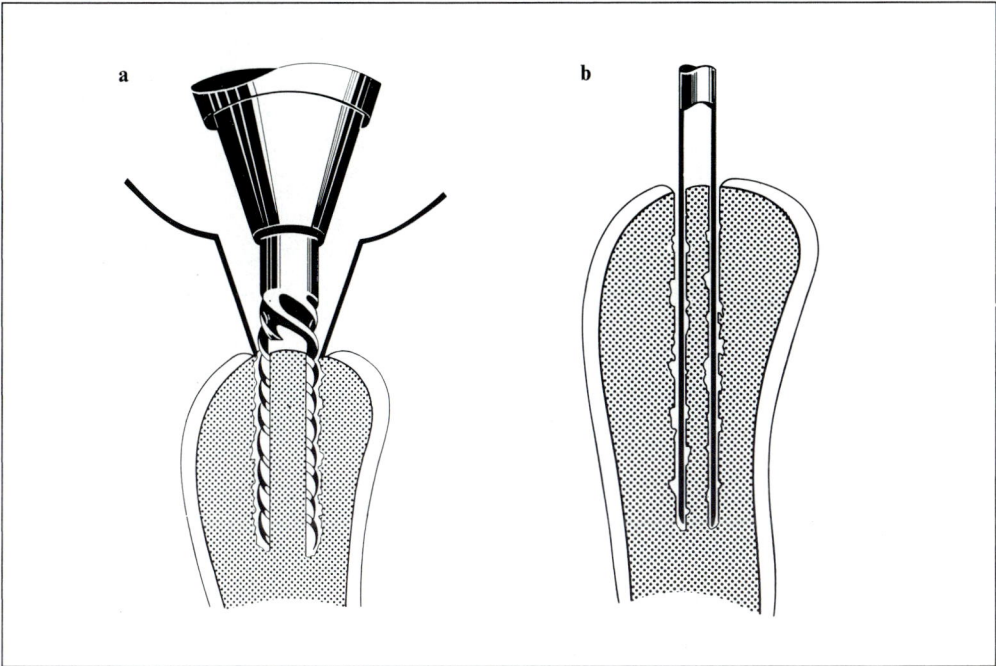

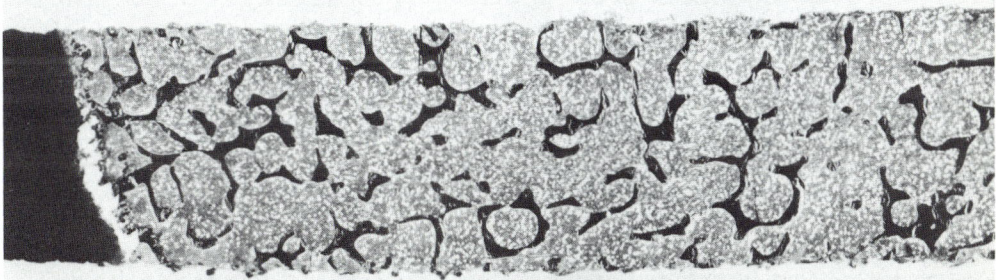

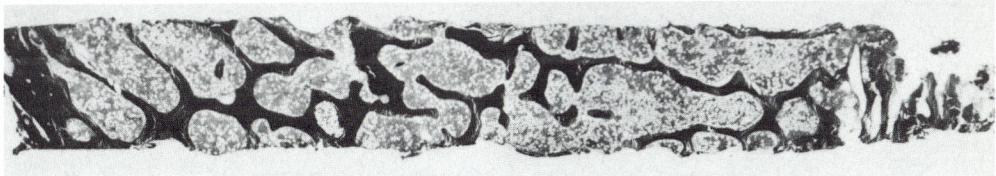

**Fig. 1.** Biopsy instruments used in this study. **a** Electric drill (Burkhardt). **b** Manual needle (Jamshidi or other).

**Fig. 2.** Representative sections of iliac crest biopsies, obtained by Burkhardt drill (**a**) and Jamshidi needle (**b**). Gomori. × 10.

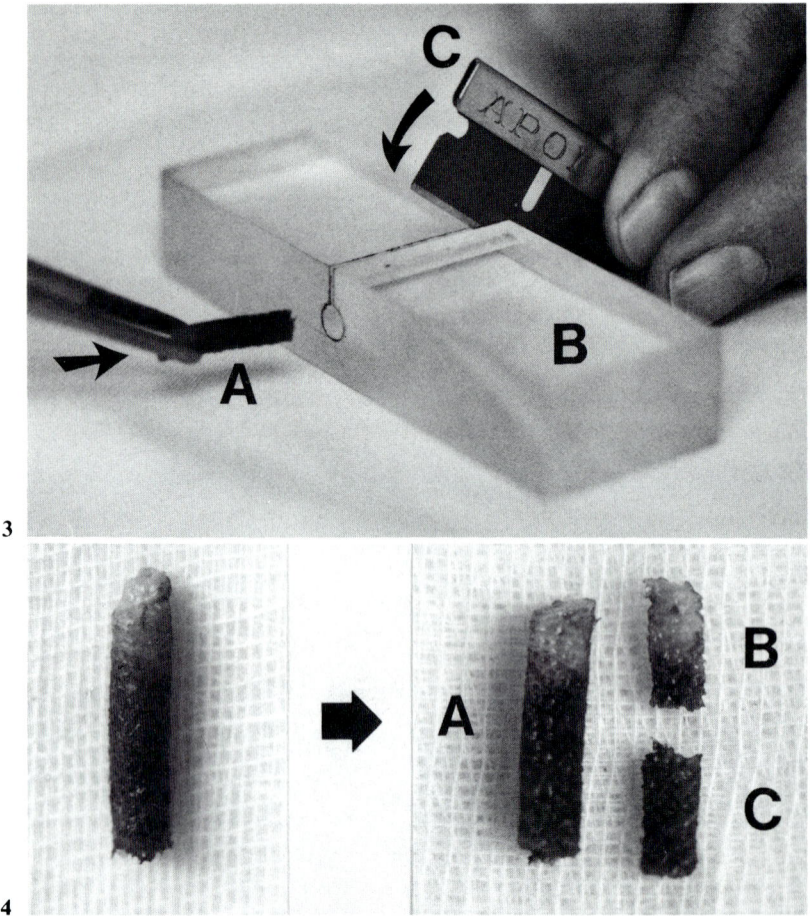

**Fig. 3.** Device for longitudinal halving of the biopsy core: the biopsy (A) is inserted sideways into the plastic holder (B) and then cut by gentle sawing action of the razor blade (C) avoiding pressure and squeezing [1].

**Fig. 4.** One longitudinally cut half (A) is embedded in methacrylate, cut surface downwards, for histology. Pieces of the second half (B, C) may be used for imprints, frozen sections and electron microscopy.

3 µm. The following stains were routinely employed: Gallamin blue-Giemsa for cytologic detail, Gomori's stain for reticulin fibres, PAS stain for glycoprotein, Ladewig's stain for calcified bone and osteoid, and the Berlin blue stain for iron. Details of the methods for processing, cutting and staining are given in *Burkhardt* [3].

In addition, the following immunohistologic methods were performed on cryostat sections of one half of unfixed, fresh frozen biopsy cores in 120 cases: (a) commercial FITC and rhodamine-labelled anti-immunoglobulins (Hyland, Behring), (b) FITC-labelled antibodies for collagen type I, II and III (kindly provided by *B. Adelmann-Grill,* Max-Planck-Institut für Biochemie, Martinsried, FRG), and peroxidase-labelled anti-immunoglobulins and rabbit-antihuman T-cell globulin (kindly provided by *G. Hoffmann-Fezer,* Institut für Hämatologie, Gesellschaft für Strahlen- und Umweltforschung, Munich, FRG) [6]. The smears or imprints made from the biopsies were stained by May-Grünwald-Giemsa's stain.

## Evaluation of Histologic Data in Relationship to Survival

A multivariate computer-based analysis of histologic data was performed and the results related to survival. 45 histologic, 12 histomorphometric [5] and 76 clinical variables were collected (list of variables in 'Appendix'). Survivals of the patients were measured from the time of the first biopsy as well as from the time of the first symptoms of disease to death or date of last contact. For statistical data analysis, selected BMPD computer programs (2D, 6D, 7D, 2F and 1L) were utilized [4], in collaboration with the MEDIS Institute, GSF, Munich. Differences between groups were evaluated for significance at the $p < 0.05$ level, for high significance at the $p < 0.01$ level. To test statistics of survival the Breslow and the Mantel-Cox tests were used [2, 7]. These tests differ in the way they emphasize the observations. The Breslow test gives greater weight to early observations and is less sensitive to late events which occur when few patients on the study remain alive. Therefore the tests are to some extent complementary.

## References

1   Bartl, R.; Burkhardt, R.; Vondracek, H.; Sommerfeld, W.; Hagemeister, E.: Rationelle Beckenkammbiopsie. Längsteilung der Proben zur Anwendung von mehreren Präparationsverfahren ohne Materialverlust. Klin. Wschr. *56:* 545–550 (1978).
2   Breslow, N.: A generalized Kruskal-Wallis test for comparing k samples subject to unequal patterns of censorship. Biometrika *57:* 579–594 (1970).
3   Burkhardt, R.: Bone marrow histology; in Catovsky, Methods in hematology. The leukemic cell, pp. 49–86 (Churchill Livingstone, Edinburgh 1981).

4    Dixon, W.J.; Brown, M.B.: BMDP-81 Biomedical Computer Programs P-Series. System, program and statistical development (University of California Press, Berkeley 1981).

5    Hennig, A.: Kritische Betrachtungen zur Volumen- und Oberflächenmessung in der Mikroskopie. Zeiss Werkzeitschr. *30:* 78–86 (1958).

6    Hoffmann-Fezer, G.; Thierfelder, S.; Pielsticker, K.; Rodt, H.: Immunohistochemical demonstration of cell surface antigens on tissue sections of lymphomas. Leuk. Res. *3:* 297–304 (1979).

7    Mantel, N.: Evaluation of survival data and two new rank order statistics arising in its consideration. Cancer Chemother. Rep. *50:* 163–170 (1966).

# 3  Structure and Function of the Normal Bone Marrow

## Structural Components

The bone marrow, one of the largest organs in the body, is situated in the cavities of the spongy bone and is composed of (1) blood vessels and nerves, (2) reticulum cells and fibres, (3) fat cells, (4) haematopoietic cells, and (5) lymphoid elements (table I) [2, 3, 9, 14].

The *blood vessels* arise from the nutrient arteries, which penetrate the bony shaft and branch in the haematopoietic tissues to form the arterial capillaries and the sinusoids. These are lined by a single layer of flat endothelial cells and constitute the outflow system for mature haematopoietic cells into the circulation. Because of the rigid bony cage the sinusoids cannot all be dilated at the same time and thus some are partially or completely collapsed. Nerve fibres accompany the marrow blood vessels. The bone marrow has no lymphatic vessels.

The *reticulum cells and fibres* form a supporting network and microenvironment for the developing blood cells. The term of 'haematopoietic inductive microenvironment' includes the concept of specific anatomic areas and cells which direct a haematopoietic stem cell to one line of differentiation or another [7, 13].

The *fat cells,* which occupy about a third of the bone marrow volume in the ilium, probably serve a supporting and filling function. The amount and distribution of fat depend on the activities of the haematopoietic cells lines (fig. 5). In case of sudden need the fat can be replaced by haematopoietic tissue very quickly. The proportion of fatty tissue increases with advancing age, at the expense of the red marrow and the bone, so that in old people it may comprise up to one half of the marrow cavities [5].

The *haematopoietic cells* lie in the spaces between the branched reticulum cells. The different cell lines which reside in the bone marrow, from the pluripotent stem cell to the differentiated end cells, are schematically illus-

**Table I.** Histomorphometry of normal bone and bone marrow – 158 bone marrow biopsies (anterior iliac crest) of normal, healthy individuals

| Variables | Mean value (SD) | Dimension |
|---|---|---|
| Haematopoietic tissue | 40 (9) | |
| Fatty tissue | 28 (8) | |
| Trabecular bone | 26 (5) | vol% |
| Osteoid | 0.3 (0.2) | |
| Sinusoids | 4.5 (2.1) | |
| Lymphocytes | 8 (7) | |
| Mast cells | 2 (1) | |
| Megakaryocytes | 8 (4) | per mm$^2$ |
| Macrophages | 16 (10) | |
| Plasma cells | 21 (18) | |
| Arteries | 3 (4) | |
| Arterioles | 26 (18) | |
| Capillaries | 101 (61) | per 100 mm$^2$ |
| Sinusoids | 1,700 (825) | |
| Osteoblastic index[1] | 5 (5) | % |
| Osteoclastic index[2] | 4 (3) | per 100 mm |

[1] Percentage of trabecular circumference covered by cuboidal osteoblasts.
[2] Number of osteoclasts per 100 mm trabecular circumference.

trated in figure 6. In bone marrow sections the erythroid precursors usually appear in small clusters, 'erythrons'. Megakaryocytes are present in relatively small numbers, but are prominent because of their size. Histotopographically 'erythrons' and megakaryocytes are associated with the central marrow sinusoids, early granulopoietic precursors are situated in proximity to the trabeculae and arterial vessels, while the more mature granulocytes are located in the central intertrabecular regions (fig. 7).

*Lymphoid elements* such as lymphoid nodules, lymphocytes and plasma cells are also encountered in the normal bone marrow. Benign lymphoid nodules were found in 2% of our 158 normal cases and in 8% of our

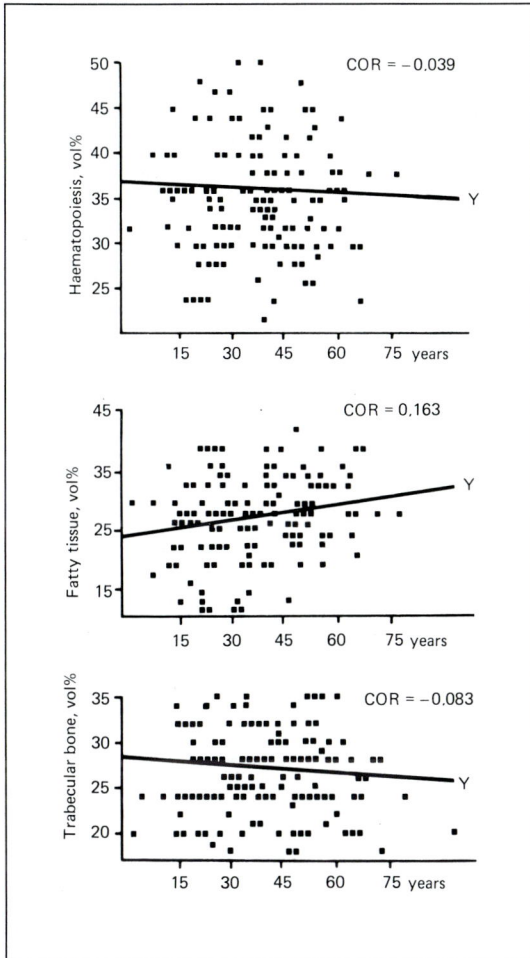

**Fig. 5.** Histomorphometric data from iliac crest biopsies, correlation with age (158 normal persons). Y = Regression line, COR = correlation factor.

overall material of 25,000 biopsies. They occur more frequently in women and in the older age groups. Together with the diffusely dispersed lympho-cytes and the fairly numerous plasma cells, mostly located around capillar-ies, these lymphoid elements indicate the immunopoietic capacity of the bone marrow [11, 12].

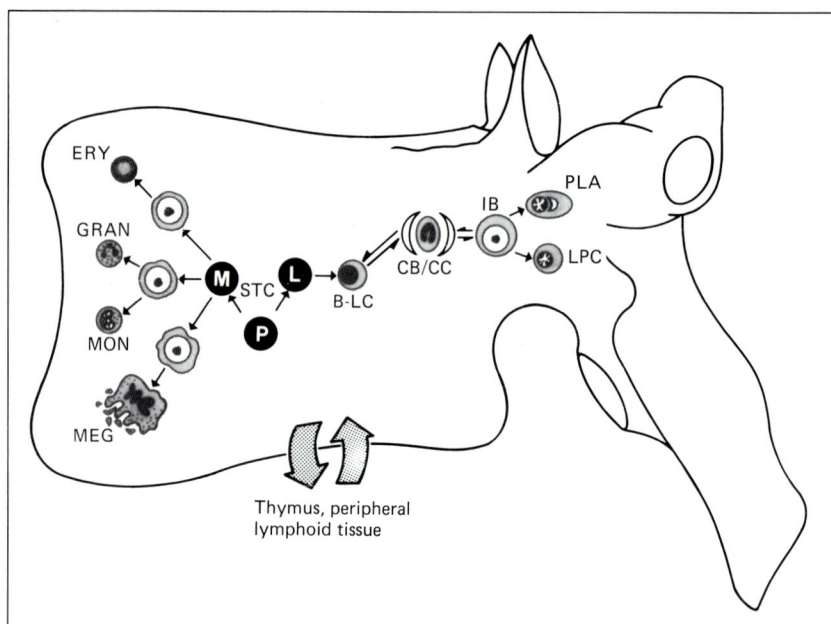

**Fig. 6.** Myeloid and lymphoid cell lines in the bone marrow: pluripotent stem cells (P) are recruited in the bone marrow for myeloid (M) and lymphoid (L) differentiation, through the mediation of cell-specific 'poietins' and of the 'haematopoietic inductive microenvironment'. The differentiation of B lymphocytes (B-LC) to functional immuno-globulin-producing cells (PLA and LPC) proceeds in the peripheral lymphatic tissues. Pluripotent cells which have migrated from the marrow and settled in the thymus differentiate into T lymphocytes. STC = Stem cells; ERY = erythropoiesis; GRAN = granulopoiesis; MON = monopoiesis; MEG = megakaryopoiesis; CB/CC = centroblastic/centrocytic cells; IB = immunoblast.

## Is the Iliac Crest Biopsy Representative of the Red Marrow at Other Sites?

In the adult, the average volume of the bone marrow is about 3,000 ml, one half of which contains red marrow [1, 8]. A large biopsy core has a volume of about 0.3 ml. So doubt arises as to whether such a small speci-men is representative of the whole organ. In addition, the variations in the proportions of fatty and haematopoietic tissues in the different parts of the skeleton must also be taken into account.

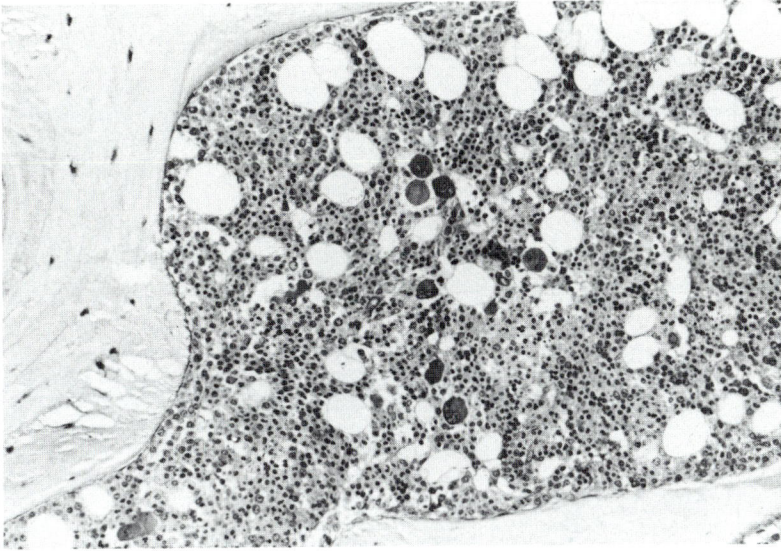

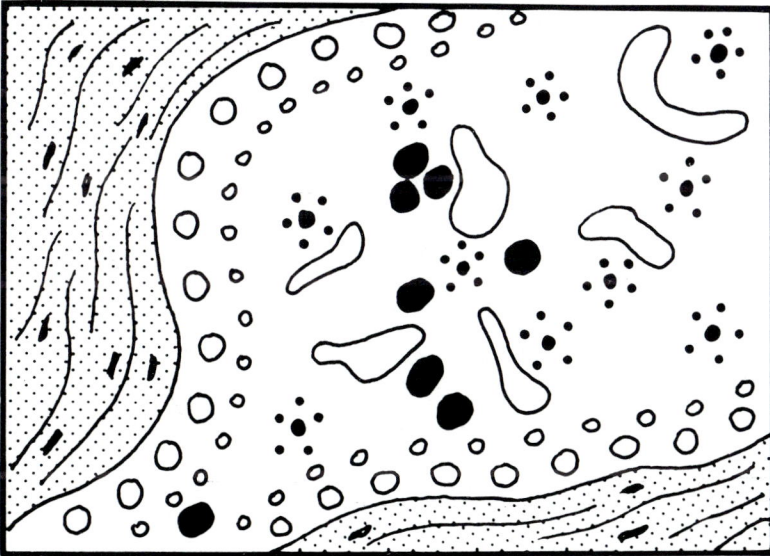

**Fig. 7.** Histotopography of normal haematopoiesis in the bone marrow: ⦂⦂ = erythropoiesis, ⬤ = megakaryopoiesis, O₀ = granulopoiesis, ⌒⌒ = sinusoid. Gallamin blue-Giemsa. × 60.

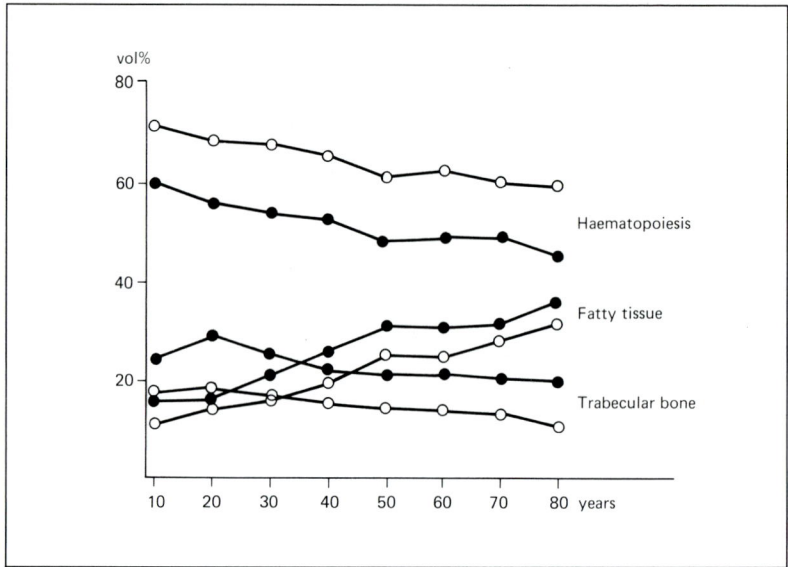

**Fig. 8.** Histomorphometric data from bone marrow biopsies, taken from the iliac crest (●) and lumbar vertebra (○), in correlation with age (150 autopsy cases, non-haematologic and non-osseous disorders) [10].

To evaluate the representativity of the iliac crest biopsy, we investigated bone marrow biopsies of 150 autopsy cases with non-haematologic and non-osseous disorders. Biopsies were taken from the sternum, the thoracic and lumbar vertebrae, and the anterior iliac crest. The median age was 52 years, the mean biopsy size 4 × 16 mm, range 6–28 mm. The volume percentages of trabecular bone, haematopoiesis and fat cells were assessed by histomorphometry, using the Zeiss integration disc II. Statistic analysis of the data showed variations between the different sites, though parallel volume deviations were observed in each case (fig. 8). The sternum and the anterior iliac crest contained more fatty tissue than the vertebrae. In a subsequent autopsy study, based on 71 cases of accidental death (median age of 48 years), parallel volume deviations were also demonstrated between the different sites of the skeleton.

Therefore, in agreement with the literature [4, 6, 10, 15], we conclude that the iliac crest biopsy may be regarded as representative of the red marrow, though there are quantitative differences between the bones containing haematopoietic tissues.

## References

1   Askanazy, M.: Knochenmark; in Handbuch der speziellen Pathologie, Anatomie und Histologie, vol. I/2, pp. 775–1014 (Springer, Berlin 1927).

2   De Bruyn, P.P.H.: Structural substrates of bone marrow function. Semin. Hematol. *18:* 179–193 (1981).

3   Burkhardt, R.: Bone marrow and bone tissue. Colour atlas of clinical histopathology (Springer, Berlin 1971).

4   Custer, R.P.; Ahlfeldt, F.E.: Studies on the structure and function of bone marrow. II. Variations in cellularity in various bones with advancing of life and their relative response to stimuli. J. Lab. clin. Med. *17:* 960–962 (1923).

5   Hartsock, R.J.; Smith, E.B.; Petty, C.S.: Normal variations with ageing of the amount of hematopoietic tissue in bone marrow from the iliac crest. Am. J. clin. Path. *43:* 326–331 (1965).

6   Kerndrup, G.; Pallesen, G.; Melsen, F.; Mosekilde, L.: Histomorphometrical determination of bone marrow cellularity in iliac crest biopsies. Scand. J. Haematol. *24:* 110–114 (1980).

7   Knospe, W.H.: Hematopoietic microenvironment: role of sinusoidal microcirculation and other stromal elements; in Aplastic anemia, pp. 95–107 (Japan Medical Research Foundation, University of Tokyo Press, Tokyo 1978).

8   Maximow, A.: Bindegewebe und blutbildende Gewebe. B. Myeloides (myeloisches) Gewebe. Das Knochenmark; in Handbuch der mikroskopischen Anatomie, vol. II/I, pp. 378–386 (Springer, Berlin 1927).

9   Mohandas, M.; Prenant, M.: Three-dimensional model of bone marrow. Blood *51:* 633–643 (1978).

10  Prechtel, K.; Kamke, W.; Osang, M.; Bartl, R.: Morphometrische Untersuchungen über altersabhängige Knochenveränderungen an Beckenkamm und Wirbelkörper post mortem. Verh. dt. Ges. Path. *60:* 356 (1976).

11  Rosse, C.; Press, O.W.: The differentiation of B and T lymphocytes from precursor cells resident in the bone marrow. Blood Cells *4:* 65–84 (1978).

12  Rywlin, A.M.; Ortega, R.S.; Dominguez, C.J.: Lymphoid nodules of bone marrow: normal and abnormal. Blood *43:* 389–400 (1974).

13  Tavassoli, M.: Studies on hemopoietic microenvironments. Exp. Hematol., Copenh. *3:* 213–226 (1975).

14  Weiss, L.; Chen, L.T.: The organization of hematopoietic cords and vascular sinuses in bone marrow. Blood Cells *1:* 617–638 (1975).

15  Xipell, J.M.; Brown, D.J.: Histology of normal bone: a computerized study in the iliac crest. Pathology *11:* 235–240 (1979).

# 4 Myeloproliferative Disorders (MPD)

## Survey of the Literature

The spectrum of MPD includes polycythaemia vera (PV), chronic myeloid leukaemia (CML), megakaryocytic myelosis (MegM) and the myelofibrosis-osteomyelosclerosis syndrome (MF/OMS). A useful unifying theory was introduced by *Dameshek* [12] in 1951 when he proposed that all the above entities be considered as a group of syndromes having in common an abnormality of the pluripotent haematopoietic stem cell [1, 14, 22]. Indeed, although different in clinical and evolutionary features, the myeloproliferative diseases have many overlapping characteristics and they may progress from one form to another [4, 7, 15, 19, 25]. Some understanding of these disorders began to dawn in 1960 with the discovery of the Philadelphia chromosome in myeloid precursors in CML [31, 35]. Subsequent studies supported the hypothesis that the spectrum of MPD reflects neoplastic pluripotent stem cell clones, with variable proliferation and differentiation abnormalities [1, 24].

The difficulty in assessing prognostic factors in MPD when considered as a single group lies in the fact that the MPD consist of well-defined clinical entities on which the previous reports on prognosis were based. The following properties of MPD may be responsible for the absence, to date, of a histologic classification:

(1) MPD are primary disorders of the bone marrow. A systematic histologic investigation of the bone marrow required appropriate biopsy techniques and optimal histologic preparations, only recently developed.

(2) In contrast to other neoplasias, there are no unequivocal cytologic characteristics which distinguish the cells in MPD from their normal counterparts in the bone marrow (at least not with current histologic techniques).

(3) Only consideration of the overall histologic and histotopographic picture permits a reliable interpretation and diagnosis. Frequently more than one haematopoietic cell line is involved and this will manifest itself in different structural characteristics and proliferation patterns. Numerous

intermediate and transitional types of MPD occur which are difficult to include in a rigid classification.

(4) The course and prognosis of MPD may be considerably altered by reactive fibrosis, which therefore must also be included in any classification system of MPD.

During the past decade combined histologic and clinical studies of specific aspects of MPD have indicated the possibility of their classification and staging. In PV, *Ellis* et al. [13] as well as *Lundin* et al. [26] gave a detailed account of the histologic findings in the bone marrow, but no prognostic factors were identified. The first histologic classification of PV was proposed by *Burkhardt* et al. [8] in 1979. MegM is recognized as a subtype of MPD, ranking close to PV in structure and prognosis [4, 13, 30, 33]. Comparative evaluation of structural and prognostic data has not been carried out in this clinical entity. CML can be divided into two histologic subgroups: the granulocytic and the megakaryo-/granulocytic types [2, 3, 6, 7, 15–17, 37]. Both types displayed the Philadelphia chromosome. We confirmed the clinical relevance of this subdivision and furthermore provided prognostic data [6, 7, 15]. MF/OMS is generally a complication of MPD and may have a considerable influence on the prognosis of the underlying disease itself [5, 6, 11, 18, 25, 27, 32, 36]. The fibrosis may reach such an extent that it completely obliterates the malignant cells which evoked it in the first place and which can no longer be identified. The stimulus for this fibrotic reaction has not yet been established definitively, though a number of possibilities has been raised [9, 10, 20–22, 28, 29, 34]. Whether MF and OMS (which is characterized by the formation of woven bone) are stages in the progression of one process or should be regarded as separate entities, is still unresolved.

## Own Observations

We investigated 584 bone marrow biopsies of 400 cases with MPD. In each case the first biopsy was performed before specific therapy was instituted. Diagnosis was made on the basis of established clinical criteria and monitored by bone marrow histology and follow-up periods of 1–10 years. The initial distribution of the patients was as follows: PV 191, CML 114, MegM 53 and MF/OMS (due to MPD of unknown origin) 42. Once the diagnosis was established, treatment with phlebotomy, busulphan or radioactive phosphorus was given according to the clinical requirements. Survival data were available for 379 cases; 114 patients had sequential biopsies. The survival curves of the clinical entities of MPD are given in figure 9. 12 histologic characteristics were assessed to investigate their predictive value in MPD.

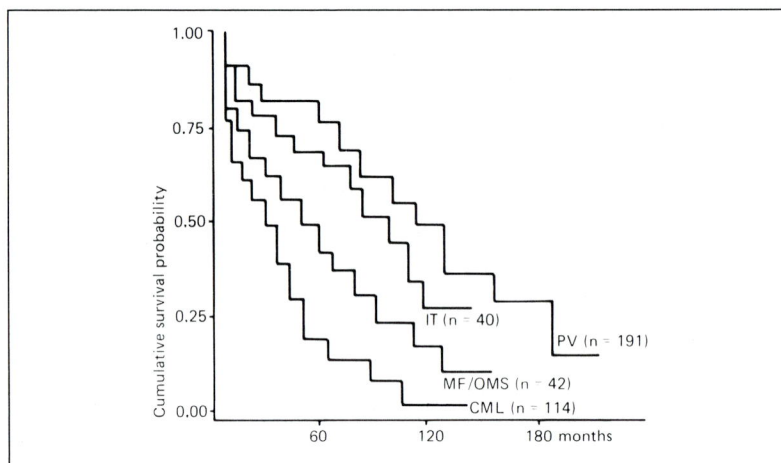

**Fig. 9.** Survival curves of MPD (clinical entities).

*Identification of Prognostic Factors in Bone Marrow Histology*

Of the 12 histologic variables analyzed, the proliferative cell line(s) proved to be the most reliable criterion and provided the most significant prognostic evaluation (table II, fig. 10, 11). The haematopoietic cell line was identified as proliferative according to cytologic, histologic and histo-topographic criteria: (1) megakaryopoietic proliferation, so-called mega-karyocytic type, with more than 20 megakaryocytes/mm$^2$ bone marrow, and exhibiting cytologic and histotopographic abnormalities, (2) erythro-poietic proliferation, so-called erythrocytic type, with erythropoietic hyper-plasia without a particular histotopographic predilection, and (3) granulo-poietic proliferation, so-called granulocytic type, with dense granulopoietic hyperplasia and broad endosteal-periarterial seams of myeloid precursors (fig. 11). Other histologic variables such as fibrosis, fatty tissue or iron also proved to be significant but not independent prognostic factors, as their occurrence was linked to the proliferative cell lines. The presence of plas-macytosis and of lymphoid nodules had no significant prognostic relevance. In the different clinical entities, survival analysis of MPD showed that increased fibre content correlated significantly with shorter survivals in PV and MegM, and with longer survivals in CML (table II). An increasing per-centage of myeloblasts in sequential biopsies signaled an unfavourable prog-nosis in CML and, to a lesser extent, in PV. A high percentage of eosinophils in bone marrow histology correlated with longer survivals in CML.

**Table II.** Prognostic factors of MPD in the bone marrow biopsy

| | Histologic criteria | Patients | Median survival months[1] | Breslow, Mantel-Cox[2] p values |
|---|---|---|---|---|
| MPD | Proliferative cell line(s) | | | 0.0001 |
| | ERY | 10 | 115 | 0.0002 |
| | ERY/GRAN | 12 | 99 | |
| | ERY/MEG | 92 | 84 | |
| | ERY/MEG/GRAN | 77 | 79 | |
| | MEG | 53 | 63 | |
| | GRAN/MEG | 62 | 27 | |
| | GRAN | 52 | 18 | |
| PV | Fibrosis | | | 0.0008 |
| | Fibrotic | 43 | 79 | 0.0007 |
| | Non-fibrotic | 78 | 132 | |
| | Fatty tissue | | | 0.6887 |
| | <5 vol% | 109 | 97 | 0.5714 |
| | ≥5 vol% | 82 | 83 | |
| | Plasma cells | | | 0.0002 |
| | Few | 96 | 130 | 0.0001 |
| | Many | 95 | 67 | |
| MegM | Cell maturity | | | 0.0001 |
| | Mature | 39 | 75 | 0.0001 |
| | Immature | 14 | 12 | |
| | Fibrosis | | | 0.1834 |
| | Fibrotic | 16 | 57 | 0.2330 |
| | Non-fibrotic | 37 | 68 | |
| | Fatty tissue | | | 0.0624 |
| | <5 vol% | 15 | 43 | 0.0510 |
| | ≥5 vol% | 38 | 78 | |
| CML | Myeloblasts | | | 0.0002 |
| | Small seams | 56 | 23 | 0.0002 |
| | Broad seams | 46 | 12 | |
| | Complete infiltration | 11 | 3 | |
| | Fibrosis | | | 0.0165 |
| | Fibrotic | 28 | 52 | 0.0054 |
| | Non-fibrotic | 86 | 29 | |
| | Fatty tissue | | | 0.0824 |
| | Absent | 80 | 20 | 0.1231 |
| | Present | 34 | 36 | |

[1] Survival time (months) was measured from the time of the biopsy to death or date of last contact.

[2] The two test statistics compare the survival curves in each variable group.

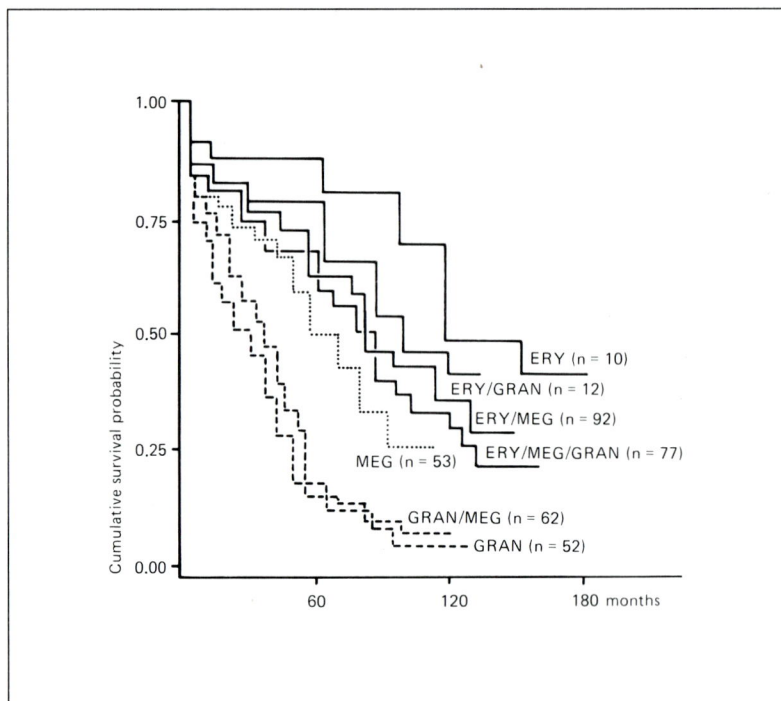

**Fig. 10.** Predictive value of bone marrow histology in MPD; grouping variable is 'proliferative cell line'.

## Histologic Classification

PV was divided into four groups according to the predominant proliferating cell line(s) in the bone marrow biopsy (table III): (1) erythro-/megakaryo-/granulocytic, (2) erythro-/megakaryocytic, (3) erythro-/granulocytic, and (4) erythrocytic. The first is the classic trilinear form of PV (fig. 12) with the following features in the biopsy: (1) hypercellularity due to hyperplasia of all the haematopoietic elements, (2) marked polymorphism, heterotopia and a striking increase of megakaryocytes, (3) hyperplasia of the sinusoids, (4) decrease of iron stores (absent in 96% of the cases), and (5) a broad spectrum in the degree of fibrosis. In the second group a marked increase in the granulocytic line did not occur (fig. 13), and the endosteal regions were occupied by the other two lines. The third group showed hyperplasia of

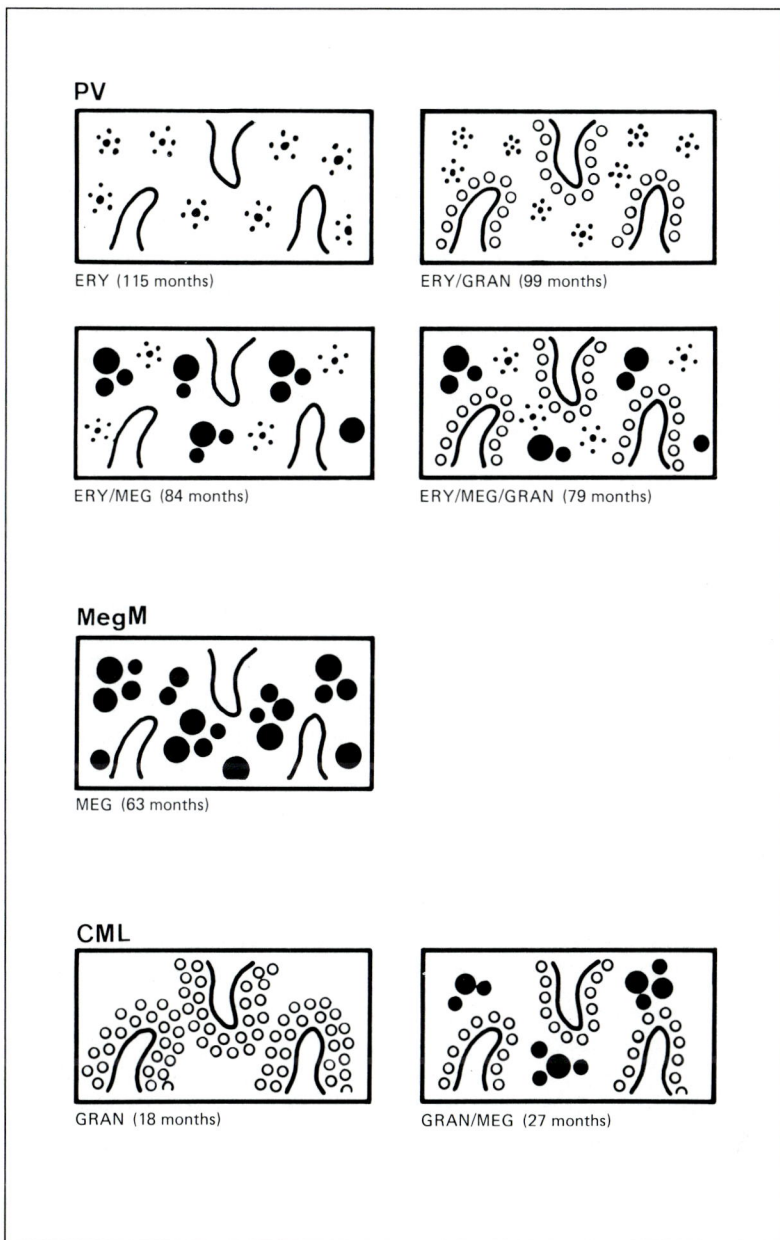

**Fig. 11.** Classification of the MPD according to the proliferative cell line(s) in the bone marrow and its prognostic relevance (median survival times).

erythroid and myeloid precursors (fig. 14), with normal numbers of mega-karyocytes. In the fourth and smallest group there was isolated hyperplasia of the erythroid cell line (fig. 15). After clinical exclusion of secondary ery-throcytosis, this group was tentatively diagnosed as PV, and the course of the disease, monitored by sequential biopsies, justified its inclusion under PV. The classification of PV into four groups on the basis of bone marrow histology had prognostic relevance (p < 0.05). The median survival was highest for the pure erythrocytic type (115 months) and lowest for the clas-sic trilinear type (79 months). As demonstrated clearly in sequential biop-sies, both the course and the metamorphosis of PV are largely influenced by the proliferating cell line(s) in the bone marrow (fig. 16). For example, the tendency to develop fibrosclerosis was observed almost exclusively in the megakaryocytic varieties. On the other hand, the kind of therapy adminis-tered, such as busulphan or radioactive phosphorus, did not carry a greater risk of inducing fibrosis. Metamorphosis of PV to terminal blast crisis was observed in 3, to other clinical entities in 16 cases (CML 5, MegM 4, NHL 4, MM 3).

Though there was some doubt in the past, idiopathic thrombo-cythaemia (IT), also called megakaryocytic myelosis *(MegM)*, is now recog-nized as a separate disease entity within the spectrum of MPD [30]. There was extreme megakaryocytic hyperplasia and polymorphism in the bone marrow, which was subdivided into mature (fig. 17, 18) and immature types (fig. 19, 20). The patients with the mature subtype had a median survival of 68 months and corresponded to the clinical entity of idiopathic thrombocythaemia. The patients with the immature (promegakaryocytic) subtype presented with thrombocytopenia, anaemia or pancytopenia and had a median survival of only 25 months. The histologic picture in sequen-tial biopsies of 5 patients with MegM demonstrated its tendency to develop into MF/OMS (fig. 21). Coarse fibrosis was first observed in proximity to clusters of polymorphous megakaryocytes.

*CML* also proved to be a heterogenous group with respect to bone marrow histology and was divided into two categories according to the proliferative cell line(s): (1) granulocytic and (2) granulo-/megakaryocytic. In both types the Philadelphia chromosome was found (assessed in 65 cases).

In the granulocytic type (fig. 22) the striking hyperplasia affected only granulopoiesis; erythropoiesis was reduced, and the mean number of mega-karyocytes was diminished. The neutrophilic form of CML was the most frequent, but predominantly eosinophilic and basophilic types were also

**Table III.** Histologic classification of MPD – 358 untreated patients at time of initial biopsy

| | ERY<br>–<br>– | ERY<br>MEG<br>– | ERY<br>MEG<br>GRAN | ERY<br>–<br>GRAN | –<br>MEG<br>– | –<br>MEG<br>GRAN | –<br>–<br>GRAN |
|---|---|---|---|---|---|---|---|
| Patients | 10 | 92 | 77 | 12 | 53 | 62 | 52 |
| Male/female | 0.7 | 0.9 | 0.6 | 0.7 | 0.6 | 0.9 | 1.8 |
| Age, median, years | 58 | 58 | 60 | 60 | 63 | 59 | 53 |
| Splenomegaly ≤ 5 cm b.c.m., %* | 20 | 33 | 22 | 36 | 31 | 26 | 36 |
| Splenomegaly > 5 cm b.c.m., % | 20 | 38 | 64 | 28 | 38 | 59 | 39 |
| Hepatomegaly ≤ 3 cm b.c.m., % | 40 | 42 | 41 | 50 | 44 | 46 | 48 |
| Hepatomegaly > 3 cm b.c.m., % | 30 | 26 | 28 | 21 | 10 | 18 | 14 |
| Anaemia (Hb < 10 g/dl), % | 10 | 8 | 8 | 8 | 35 | 35 | 35 |
| Polyglobulia (Hb > 16 g/dl), % | 70 | 68 | 56 | 65 | 0 | 0 | 0 |
| Leukopenia (< 4 × $10^9$/l), % | 10 | 15 | 2 | 0 | 16 | 0 | 0 |
| Leukocytosis (> 10 × $10^9$/l), % | 30 | 35 | 66 | 64 | 50 | 47 | 34 |
| Leukocytosis (> 50 × $10^9$/l), % | 0 | 0 | 0 | 8 | 2 | 40 | 60 |
| Thrombopenia (< 200 × $10^9$/l), % | 40 | 32 | 30 | 46 | 8 | 36 | 58 |
| Thrombocytosis (> 400 × $10^9$/l), % | 0 | 15 | 22 | 18 | 15 | 30 | 8 |
| Thrombocytosis (> 800 × $10^9$/l), % | 0 | 9 | 9 | 0 | 60 | 15 | 0 |
| Erythroblasts, peripheral, % | 10 | 19 | 25 | 0 | 8 | 28 | 12 |
| LAP decreased, % | 0 | 8 | 4 | 0 | 53 | 42 | 68 |
| LAP increased, % | 100 | 60 | 68 | 75 | 20 | 10 | 4 |
| Haematopoietic tissue, vol% | 50 (10) | 51 (16) | 60 (21) | 60 (22) | 36 (21) | 68 (20) | 73 (12) |
| Fatty tissue, vol% | 7 (8) | 10 (9) | 5 (4) | 4 (4) | 25 (10) | 5 (6) | 2 (3) |
| Sinusoids, vol% | 9 (3) | 8 (3) | 7 (3) | 8 (4) | 7 (3) | 6 (4) | 2 (1) |
| Trabecular bone, vol% | 27 (4) | 25 (9) | 24 (8) | 23 (5) | 24 (4) | 22 (8) | 20 (5) |
| Megakaryocytes per mm² marrow | 9 (5) | 20 (9) | 40 (96) | 9 (5) | 204 (254) | 98 (56) | 5 (4) |
| Lymphoid nodules, % | 20 | 26 | 25 | 15 | 18 | 18 | 4 |

ERY = Erythropoiesis, MEG = megakaryopoiesis, GRAN = granulopoiesis; b.c.m. = below costal margin; %* = percentage in each histologic group; numbers in parentheses = standard deviations; LAP = leukocyte alkaline phosphatase.

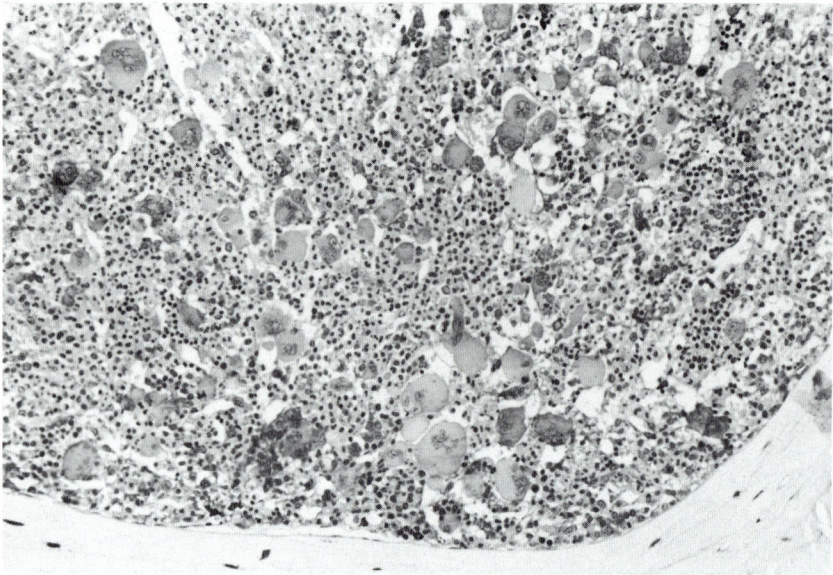

12

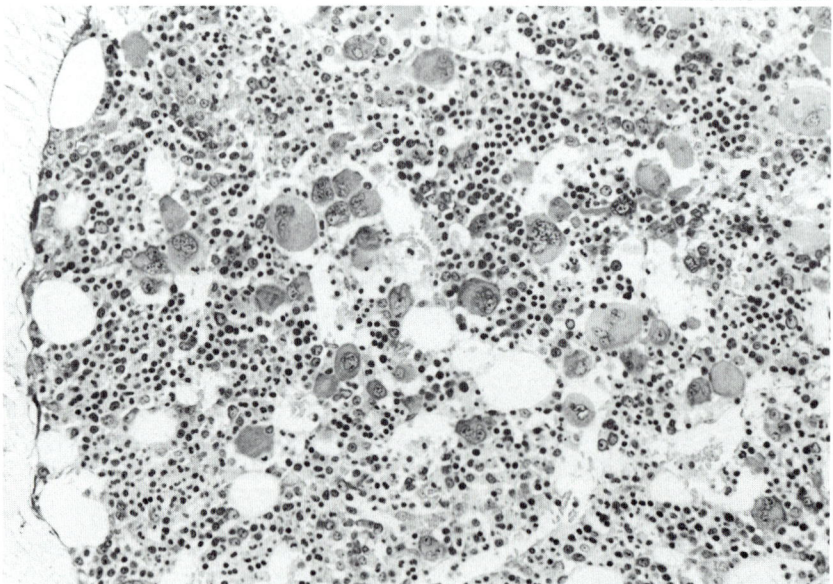

13

**Fig. 12.** PV, erythro-/megakaryo-/granulocytic type. Giemsa. ×60.
**Fig. 13.** PV, erythro-/megakaryocytic type. Giemsa. ×60.

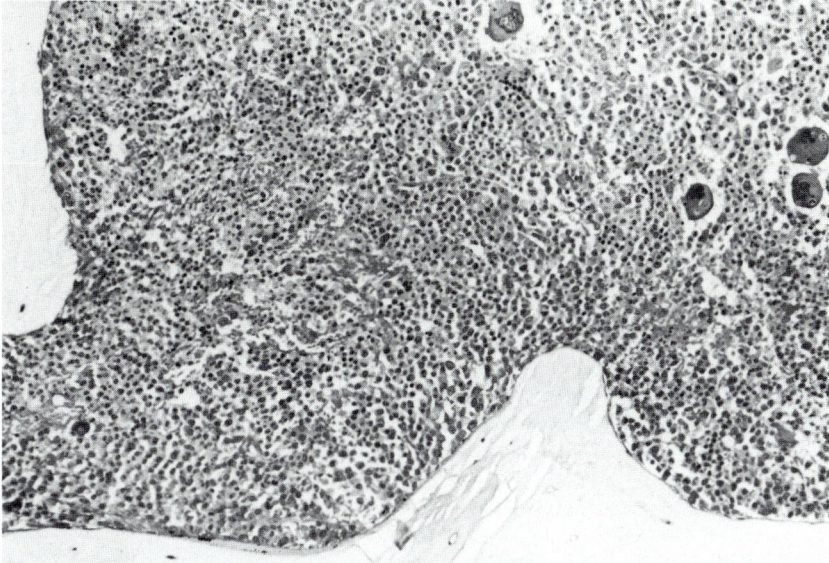

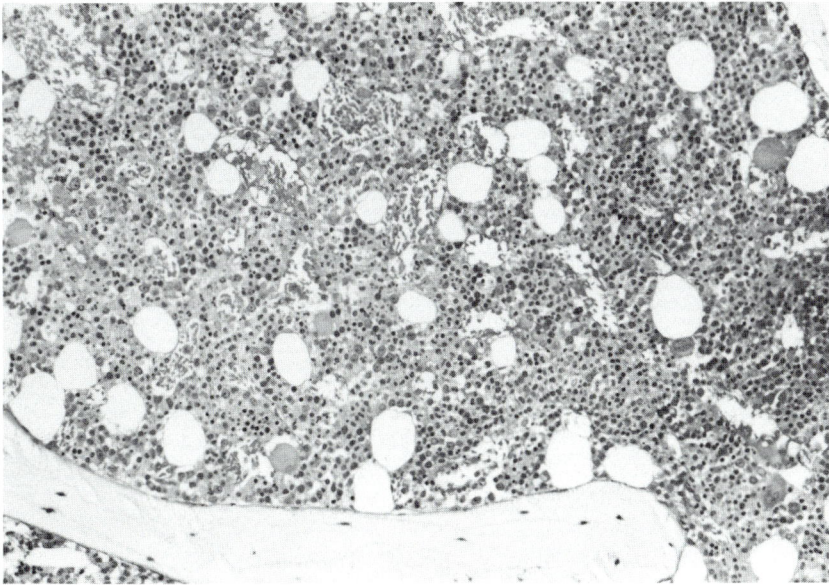

**Fig. 14.** PV, erythro-/granulocytic type. Giemsa. × 60.
**Fig. 15.** PV, erythrocytic type. Giemsa. × 60.

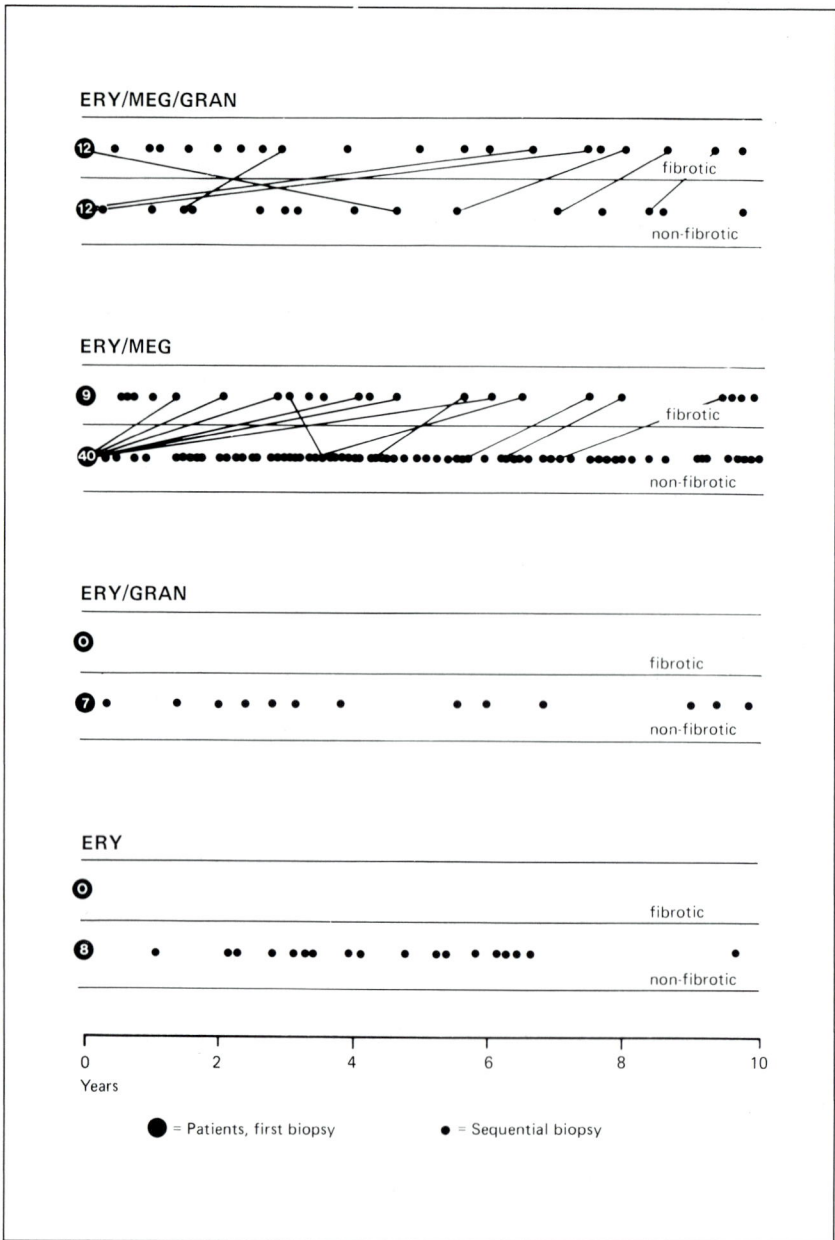

**Fig. 16.** Fibrotic transformation in the different histologic types of PV, 88 patients with sequential biopsies.

observed. Seams of myeloblasts and promyelocytes in the paratrabecular areas, usually with an abrupt transition to mature granulocytes in the central regions, may be regarded as the specific growth pattern in this type of CML. Reticulin fibres were normal or only slightly increased, but fat cells were markedly reduced.

In the mixed type (fig. 23) there were quantitative and qualitative alterations of megakaryopoiesis as shown by the occurrence of highly polymorphic, heterotopic as well as immature megakaryocytes. The megakaryocytes, single and in clusters, were usually situated in the central intertrabecular areas and close to the hyperplastic sinusoids, frequently in their lumina. A variable increase in fibres was always present, particularly adjacent to megakaryocytic clusters and arterial vessels. An increase in plasma cells and mast cells was found in both histologic types of CML.

This histologic classification has prognostic value, though it is statistically significant only in the Breslow test ($p < 0.05$). Patients with the granulocytic type of CML had a median survival of 18 months, those with the mixed type of 27 months. The practical value of this histologic classification emerged in our follow-up studies. The assessment of sequential biopsies clearly demonstrated that transformation to myelofibrosis occurred only in the mixed type, and metamorphosis to a terminal blast crisis was seen predominantly in the granulocytic type, which may be the main reason for its less favourable prognosis (fig. 24, 25). Expanding myeloblastic seams in sequential biopsies proved to be a reliable sign of imminent blast crisis (fig. 26). Metamorphosis to other diseases was observed in 6 cases (MegM 3, NHL 2, MM 1).

### Myelofibrosis-Osteomyelosclerosis Syndrome (MF/OMS)

Since fibrosis itself has a considerable influence on the prognosis of the primary disease, its clinical and prognostic relevance has been analyzed in this study (fig. 27, 28). Transformation to MF/OMS was observed in about 50% of the patients with MPD (61% in MegM, 52% in PV, 46% in CML). The basic myeloproliferative process was known in 87% of the patients with MF/OMS; in 13% the underlying myeloproliferative disorder could not be identified (table IV).

The histologic picture of myelofibrosis is characterized by a diffuse network of coarse fibres (collagen type III) which divide the marrow cavities into small compartments (fig. 29–31). Clusters of polymorphous megakaryocytes are surrounded by fibrotic tissue and are located close to the sclerotic walls of ectatic sinusoids (fig. 30, 32). Oedema and dislodged plate-

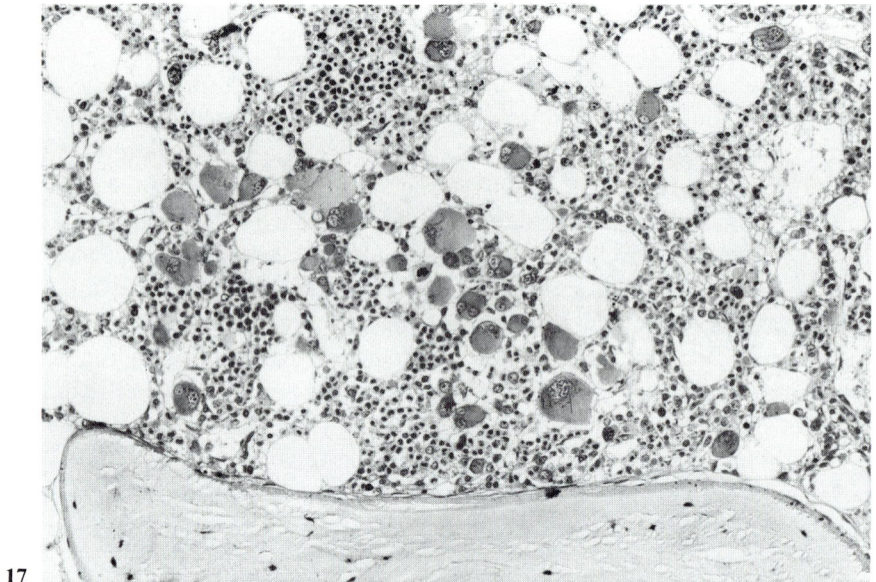

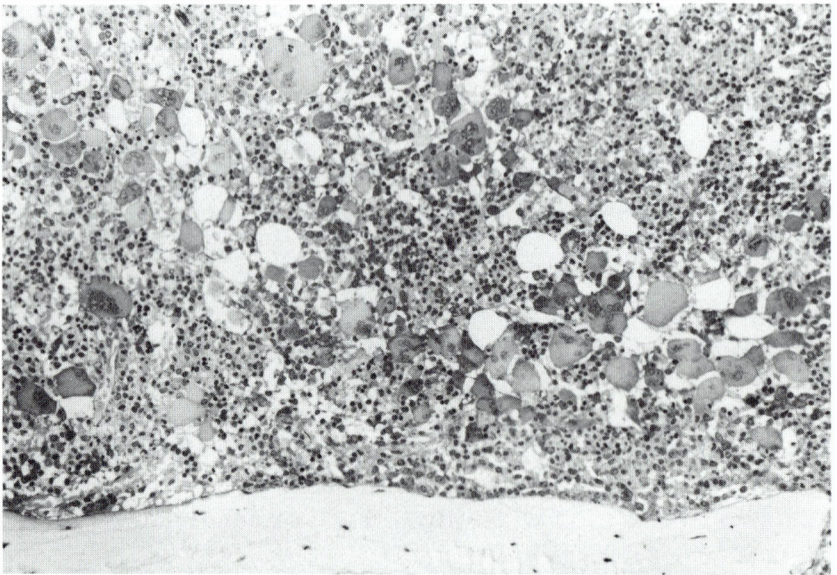

**Fig. 17.** MegM, mature type. Giemsa. × 60.
**Fig. 18.** MegM, mature type with marked granulopoietic activity. Giemsa. × 60.

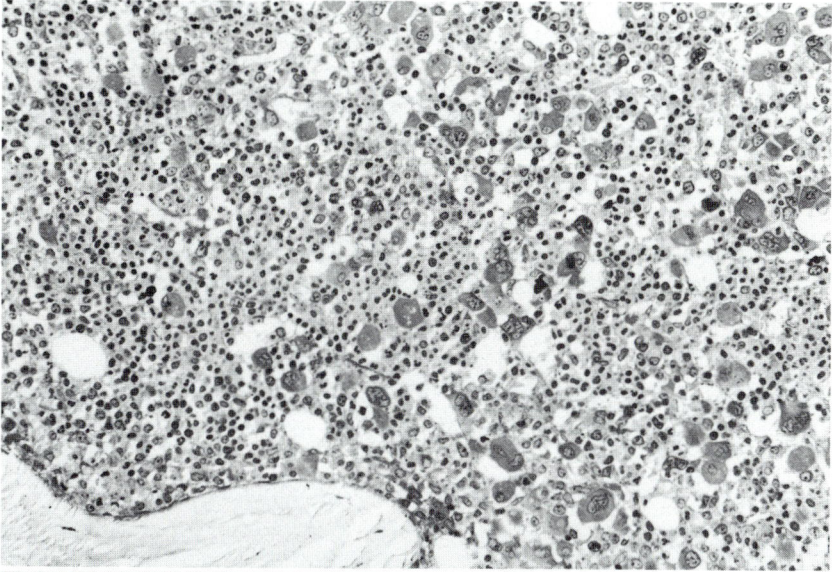

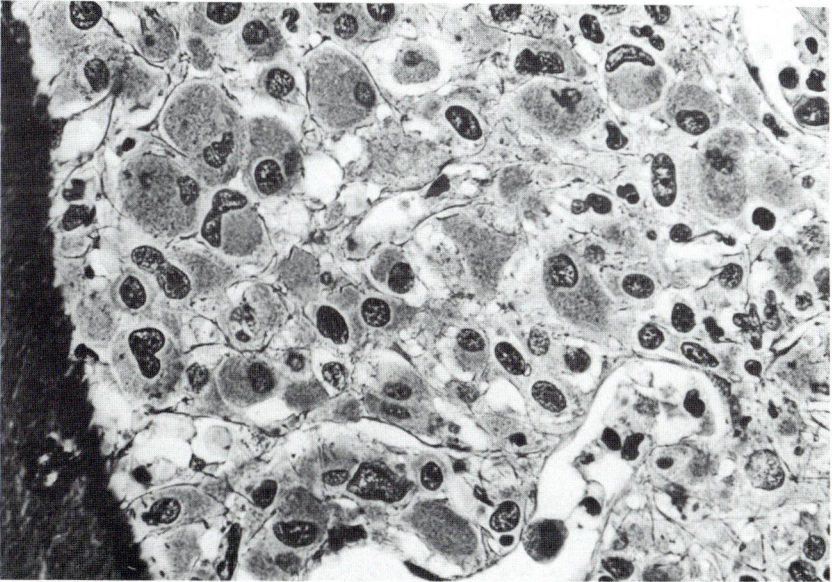

**Fig. 19.** MegM, immature type. Giemsa. × 60.
**Fig. 20.** MegM, immature type. Gomori. × 250.

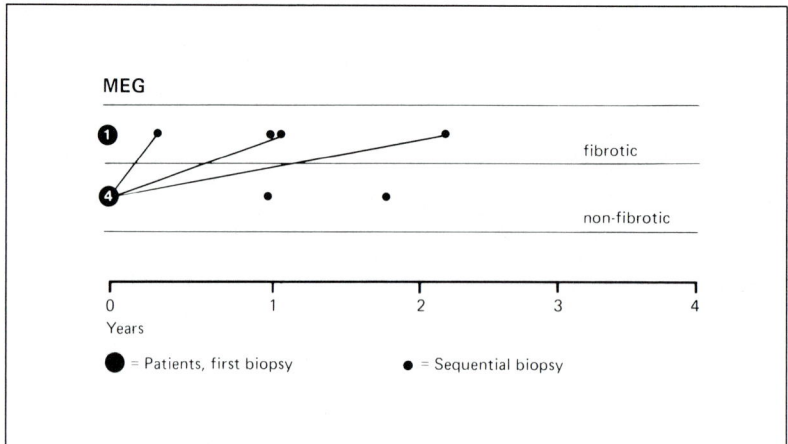

**Fig. 21.** Fibrotic transformation in MegM, 5 patients with sequential biopsies.

lets are found in the interstitial spaces (fig. 33). Morphologic signs of inflammation such as infiltrations of lymphocytes, plasma cells and mast cells are always present. Haematopoiesis is considerably diminished till finally there is complete replacement by fibrosis. The histologic diagnosis of OMS is made when woven bone is present in addition to the histologic findings described above (fig. 29, 34). This primitive, poorly mineralized bone is randomly interwoven to a variable extent with the fibrous tissue which occupies the intertrabecular cavities of lamellar bone. The content of fat cells is usually higher than in MF, in contrast to the greater decrease in haematopoietic tissue (table IV). Histotopographically, striking variations were observed in MF/OMS; however, their clinical and prognostic relevance remains unclear (fig. 35, 36).

Though there is a close pathogenic relationship between MF and OMS, there are differences in the clinical course and prognosis which is more favourable in OMS than in MF (75%/50% survival times of 21/51 and 5/50 months, respectively). The median time from the first symptoms to the biopsy was 5 years in MF and 4 years in OMS. On the basis of follow-up studies we were able to demonstrate that OMS is not necessarily a later or more advanced stage of MF; the two types should be regarded as qualitatively and quantitatively different modes of stromal reaction to the myelo-

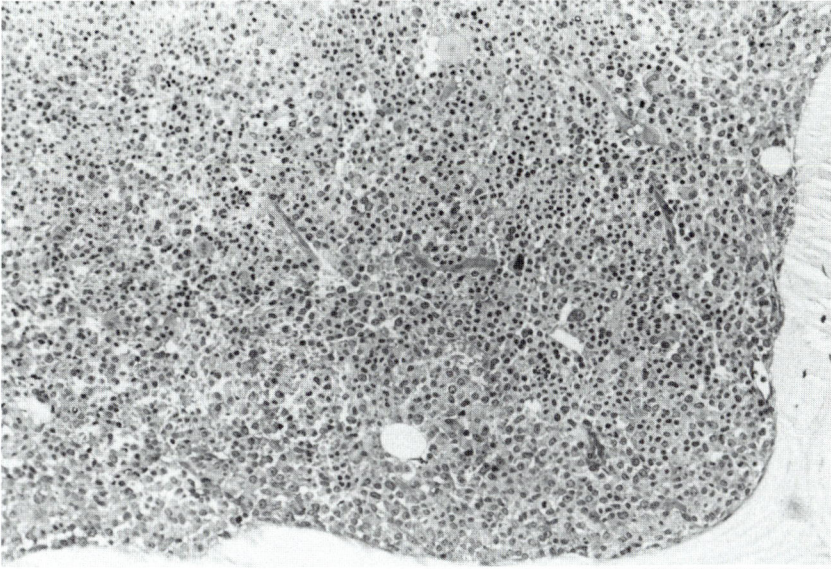

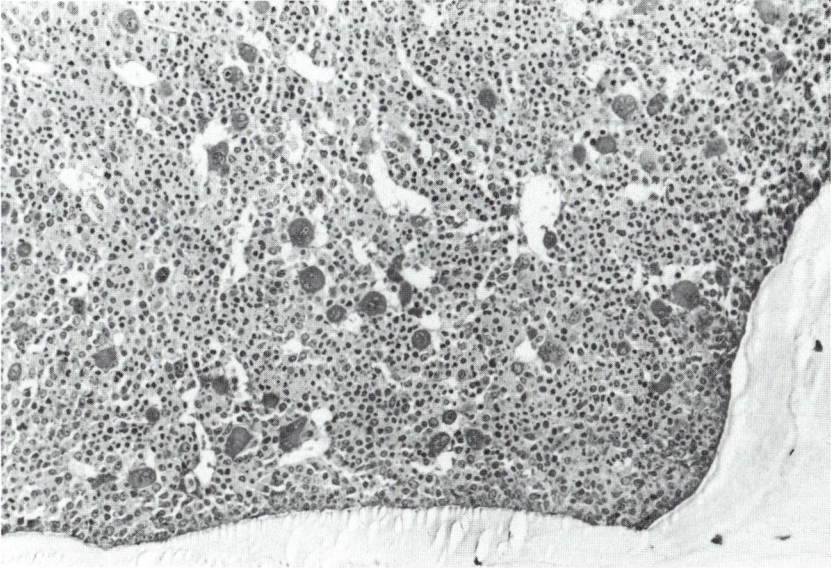

**Fig. 22.** CML, granulocytic type. Gallamin blue-Giemsa. × 60.
**Fig. 23.** CML, granulo-/megakaryocytic type. Gallamin blue-Giemsa. × 60.

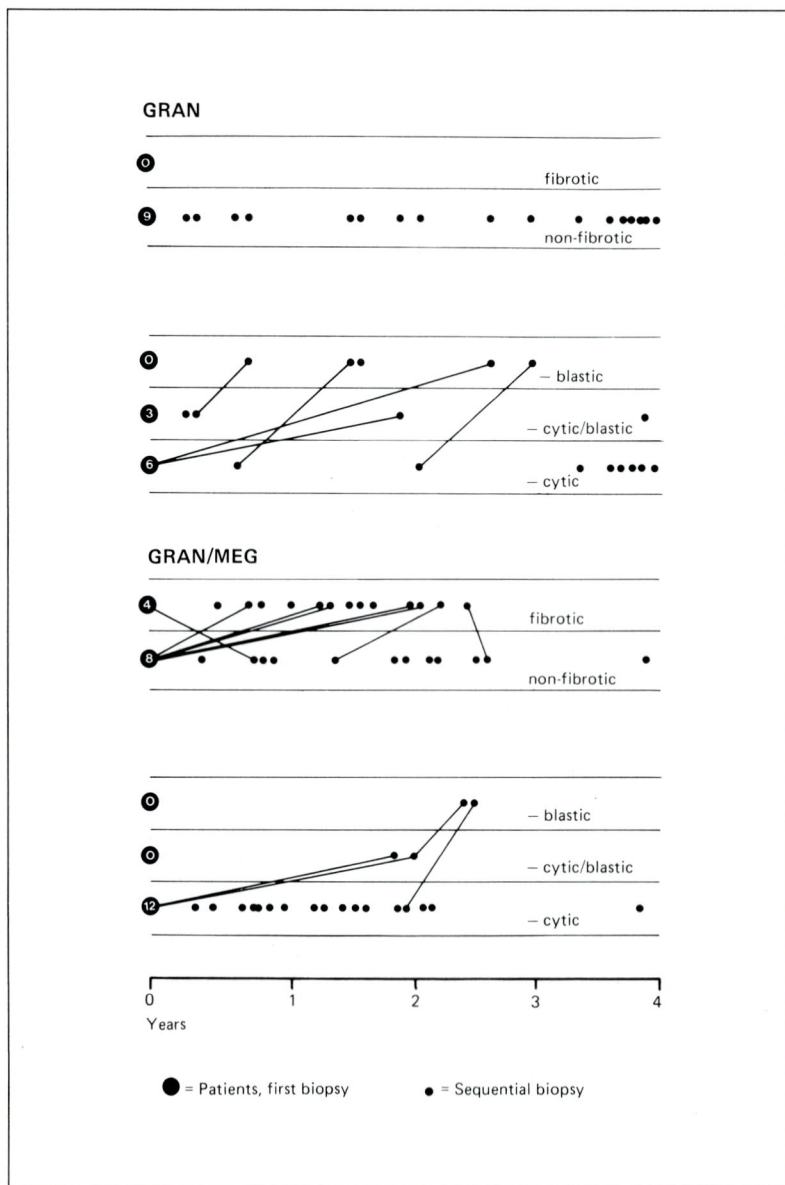

**Fig. 24.** Fibrotic and blastic transformation in the different histology types of CML, 21 patients with sequential biopsies.

**Fig. 25.** Metamorphosis of both histologic types of CML. F = MF/OMS; B = blastic crisis; A = aplastic crisis.

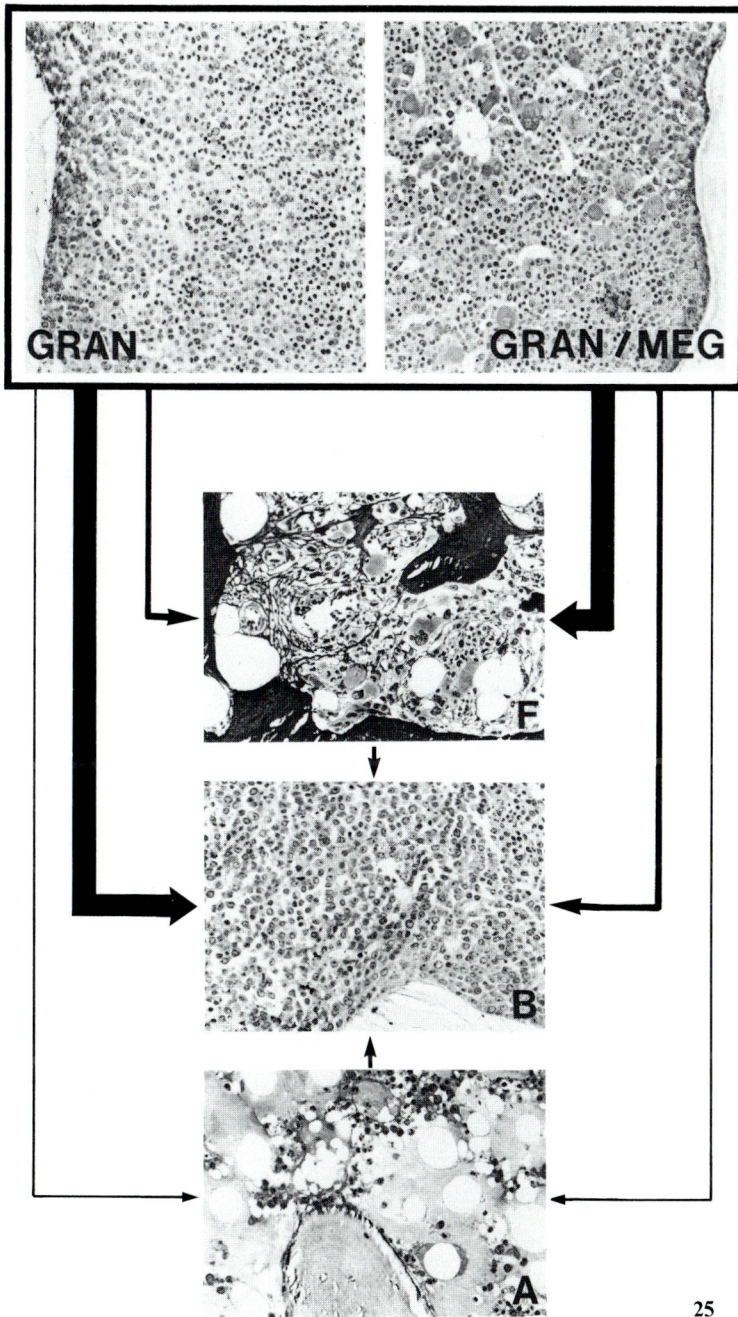

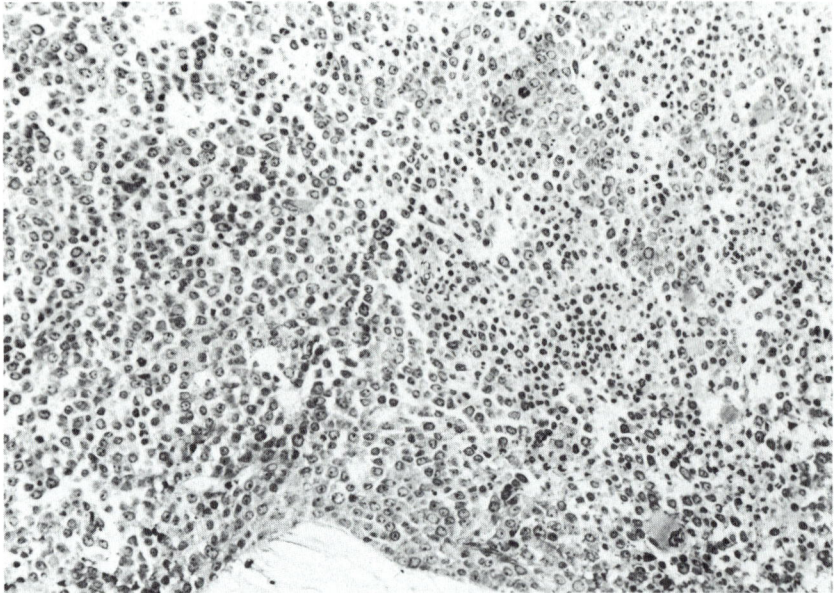

26

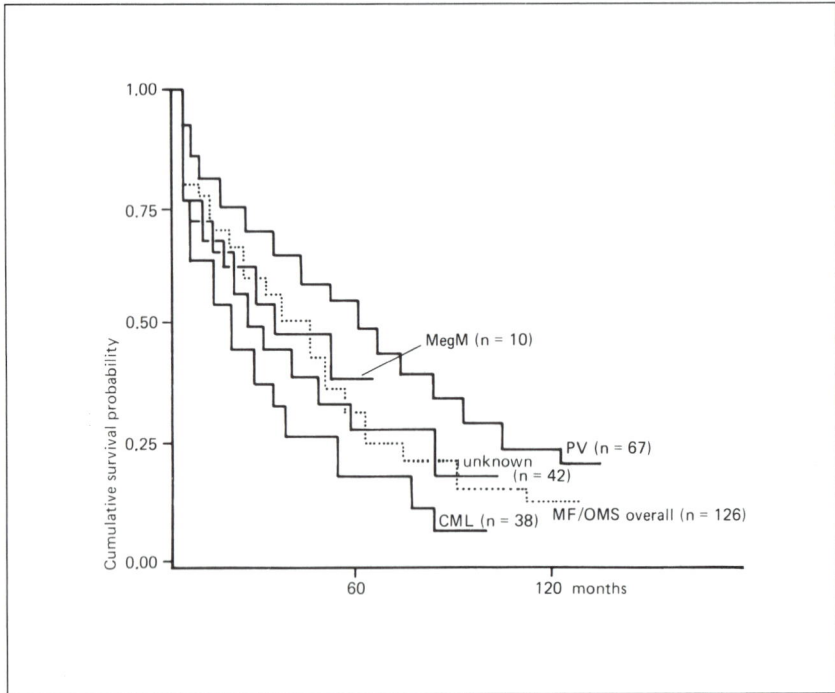

27

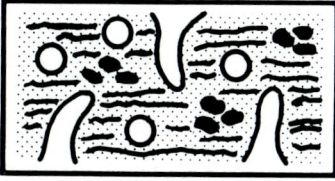

Myelofibrotic (50 months)

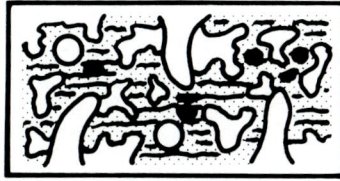

Osteomyelosclerotic (51 months)

28

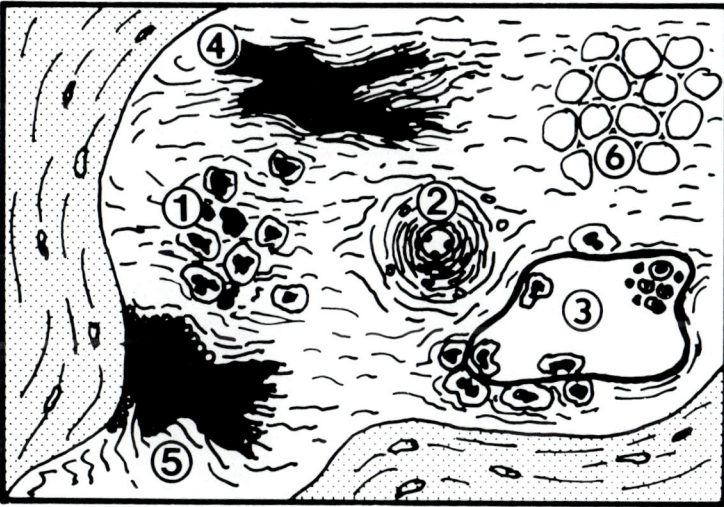

29

**Fig. 26.** CML, granulocytic type. Transition to blastic crisis with a high content of myeloblasts and promyelocytes. Giemsa. × 60.

**Fig. 27.** Predictive value of the underlying MPD in MF/OMS.

**Fig. 28.** Patterns of MF/OMS in the bone marrow histology and their prognostic relevance (median survival time).

**Fig. 29.** Diagnostic criteria of MF/OMS in the bone marrow biopsy: 1 = clusters of megakaryocytes; 2 = perivascular fibrosis; 3 = ectatic sinusoids with precursors of erythro- and megakaryopoiesis in the lumen; 4 = woven bone in the centre of the marrow space; 5 = woven bone in apposition to the lamellar bone; 6 = patchy areas of fatty tissue.

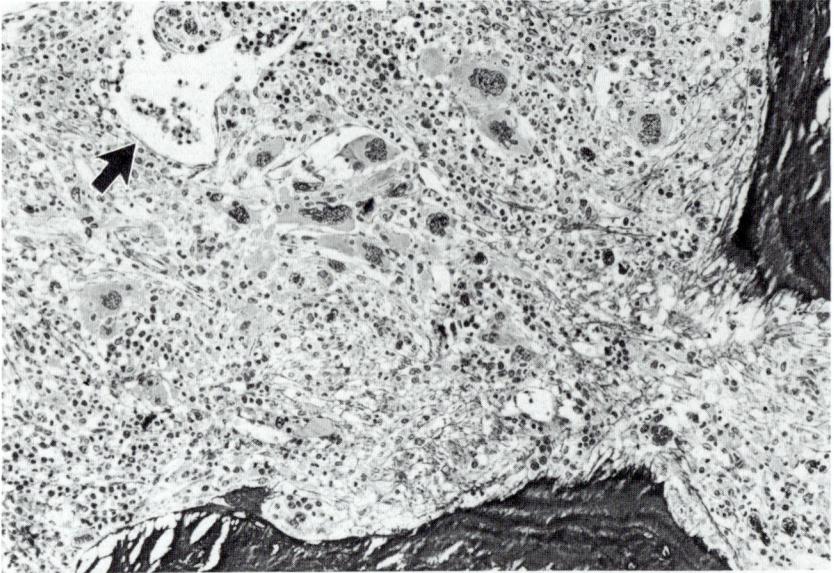

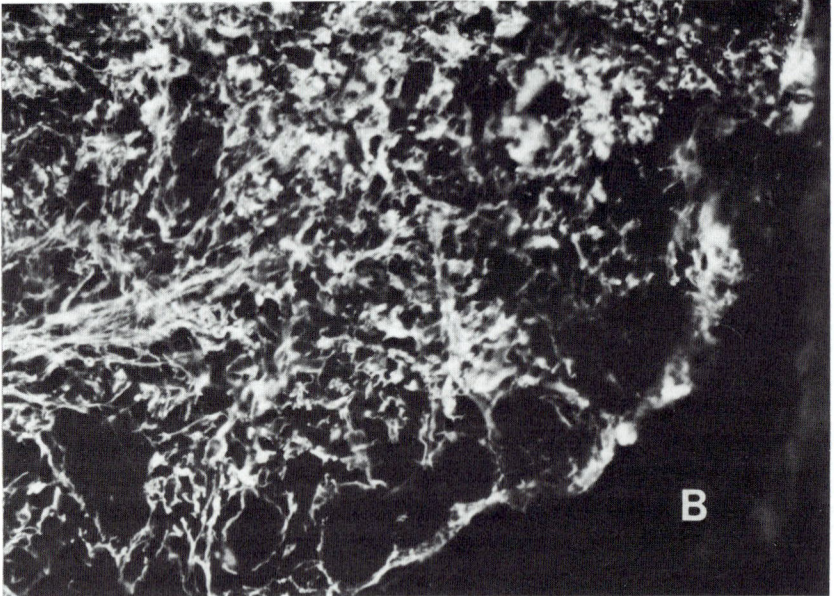

**Fig. 30.** Myelofibrosis syndrome on the basis of CML, granulo-/megakaryocytic type. Erythroid precursors in the lumen of an ectatic sinusoid (arrow). Gomori. × 100.

**Fig. 31.** Immunohistologic demonstration of collagen type III, in myelofibrosis on the basis of MegM. B = Trabecular bone. Frozen bone marrow section, FITC, anti-collagen type III. × 100.

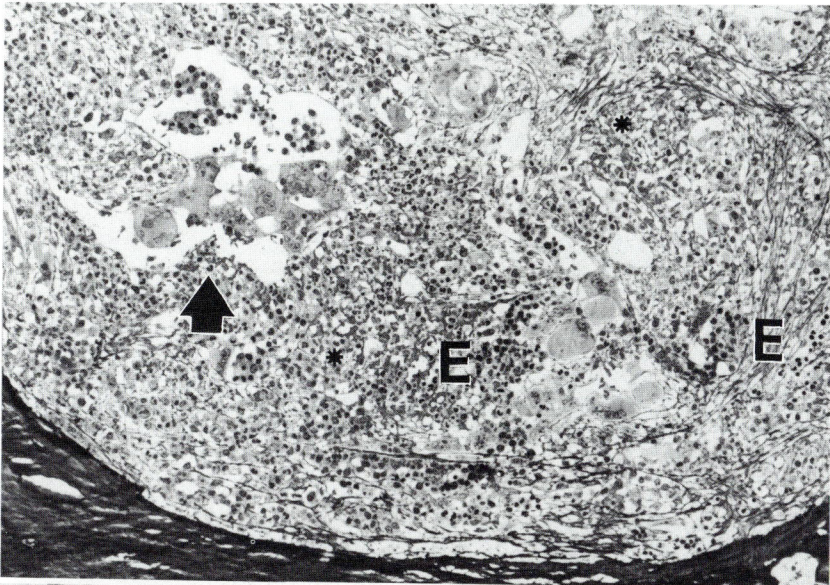

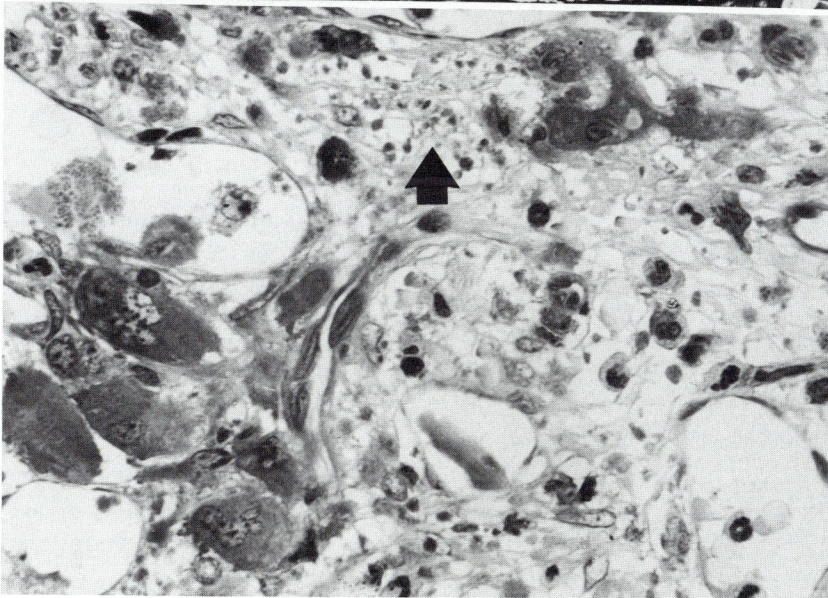

**Fig. 32.** MF on the basis of MegM, with atypical polymorphic megakaryocytes, partly lying in the lumen of ectatic sinusoids (arrow); E = erythropoiesis with maturation inhibition; * = extravasates of erythrocytes. Gomori. × 250.

**Fig. 33.** MF on the basis of CML. Dislodged platelets (arrow) between atypical, heterotopic megakaryocytes. Giemsa. × 400.

**Table IV.** Histologic classification of MF/OMS – 135 patients

|  | MF | OMS |
|---|---|---|
| Patients | 75 | 60 |
| Male/female | 0.6 | 1.0 |
| Age, median, years | 66 | 56 |
| Osteoporosis (X ray), % | 12 | 9 |
| Osteosclerosis (X ray), % | 2 | 41 |
| Splenomegaly < 5 cm b.c.m., % | 15 | 20 |
| Splenomegaly > 5 cm b.c.m., % | 65 | 76 |
| Hepatomegaly < 4 cm b.c.m., % | 48 | 53 |
| Hepatomegaly > 4 cm b.c.m., % | 28 | 25 |
| Anaemia (Hb < 10 g/dl), % | 48 | 39 |
| Leukopenia (< 4 × $10^9$/l), % | 20 | 10 |
| Leukocytosis (> 10 × $10^9$/l), % | 40 | 45 |
| Thrombopenia (< 200 × $10^9$/l), % | 38 | 34 |
| Thrombocytosis (> 400 × $10^9$/l), % | 34 | 22 |
| Erythroblasts, peripheral, % | 70 | 68 |
| LAP decreased, % | 12 | 15 |
| LAP increased, % | 39 | 32 |
| ESR > 50 mm/h, % | 58 | 14 |
| Haematopoietic tissue, vol% | 45 (19) | 22 (16) |
| Fatty tissue, vol% | 9 (9) | 16 (14) |
| Fibrotic tissue, vol% | 6 (8) | 5 (4) |
| Sinusoids, vol% | 8 (6) | 7 (5) |
| Trabecular bone, vol% | 24 (5) | 40 (14) |
| Osteoid, vol% | 1 (2) | 6 (7) |
| Woven bone, vol% | 0 | 16 (14) |
| Megakaryocytes per $mm^2$ marrow | 85 (61) | 41 (30) |
| Lymphoid nodules, % | 20 | 10 |

b.c.m. = Below costal margin; number in parentheses = standard deviations; LAP = leukocyte alkaline phosphatase.

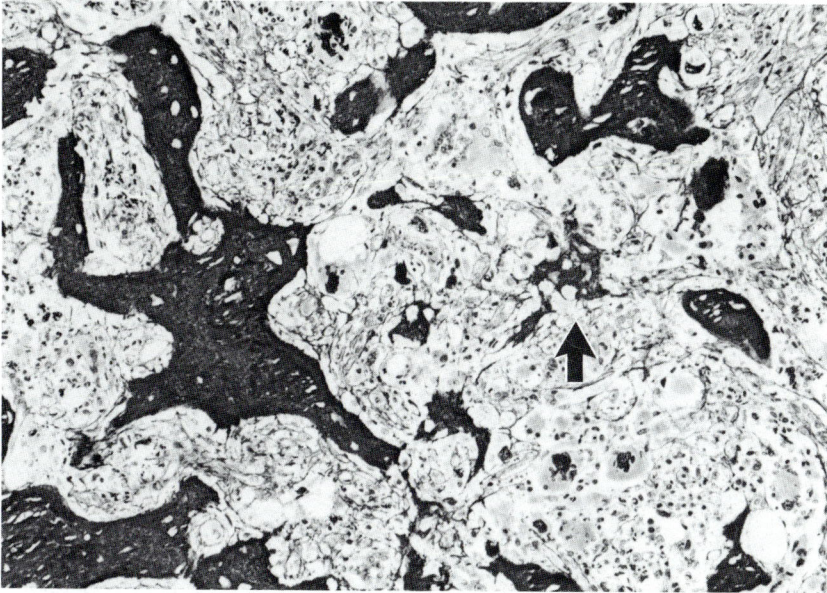

**Fig. 34.** Osteomyelosclerosis syndrome. Production of woven bone (arrow) between megakaryocytic clusters. Gomori. × 100.

proliferation. A highly significant connection was evident between the presence of proliferating megakaryocytes and the development of fibrosis. Therapy with busulphan or radioactive phosphorus did not increase the risk of developing fibrosis (fig. 37): 78% of the patients with MF/OMS had no cytostatic therapy before the biopsy. On the other hand, it is highly probable that these agents suppress megakaryopoiesis and thus diminish the main stimulus for fibroblast proliferation and production of fibrosis.

**Implications for Medical Practice**

During the past decade several large series have demonstrated the clinical value of bone marrow biopsy for diagnosis and monitoring of various clinical entities within the MPD. In this study we have shown that bone marrow histology is required in order accurately to classify the main groups and subgroups according to those histologic parameters that have prognos-

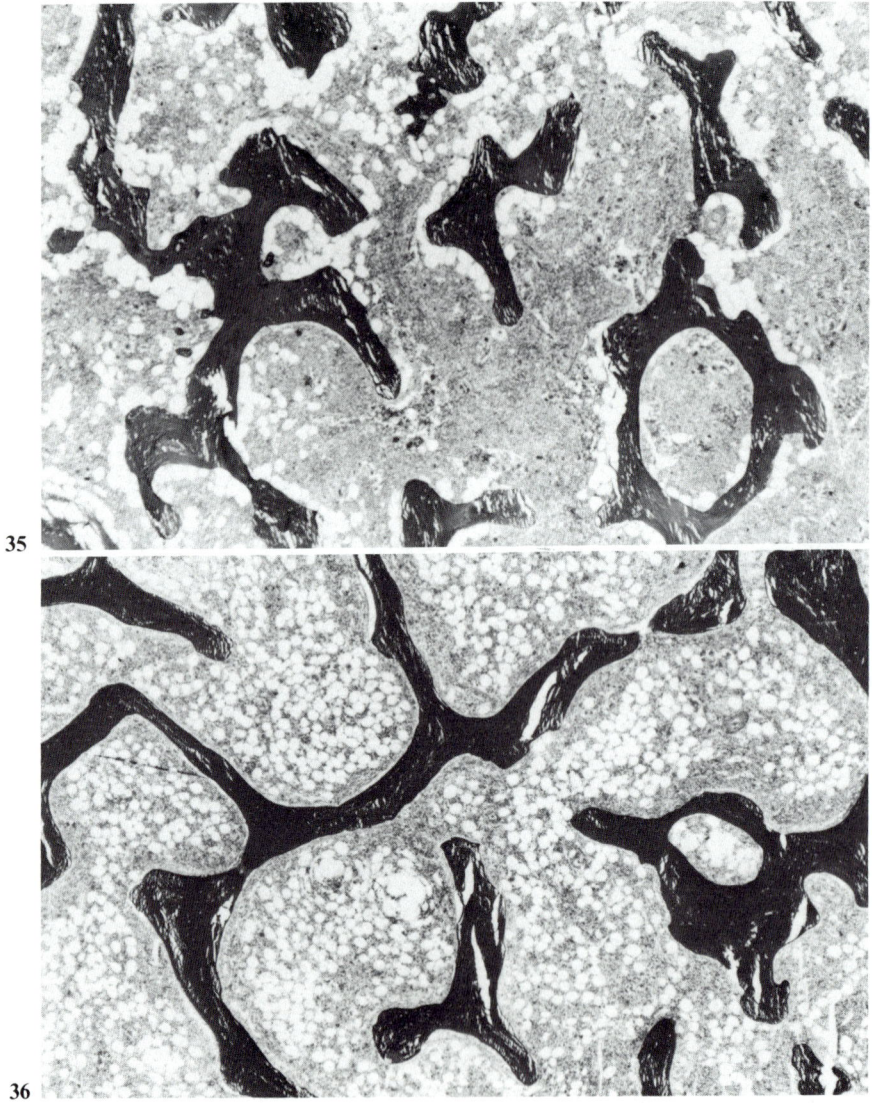

**Fig. 35.** Endosteal seams of fatty tissue in MF. Gomori. × 100.
**Fig. 36.** Central localisation of fatty tissue in MF. Gomori. × 100.

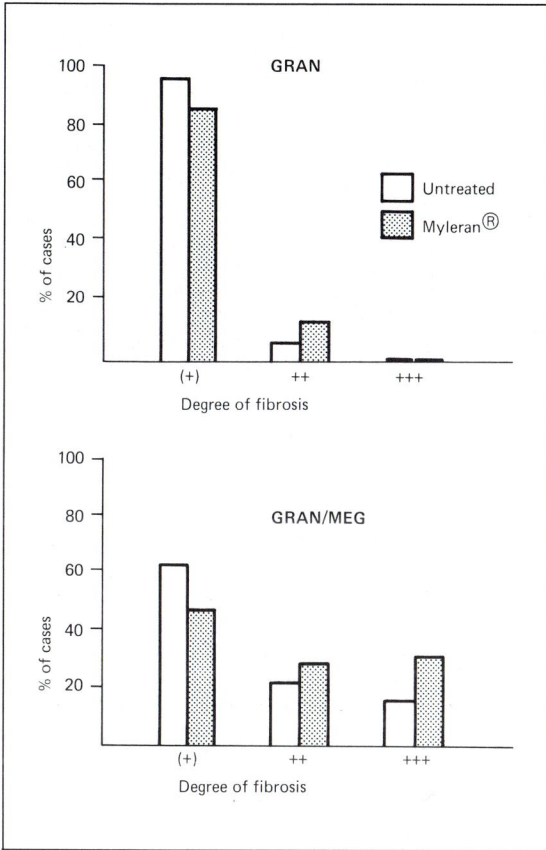

**Fig. 37.** Frequency of fibrotic transformation in CML. Variables are 'mode of thera-py' and 'histologic subtype'.

tic relevance. The most reliable and prognostically the most significant parameter to emerge, after grouping the whole spectrum of MPD together, proved to be the proliferative cell line(s) in the bone marrow. An erroneous interpretation of the myeloproliferation, caused by histotopographic varia-tions within the same biopsy (fig. 38), can be excluded by assessment of at least five marrow spaces (about 30 mm$^2$ bone marrow area).

On the basis of this histologic parameter we propose a classification system which has both clinical and prognostic relevance (table V) and may be summarized as follows: PV is subdivided into four groups: (1) eryth-

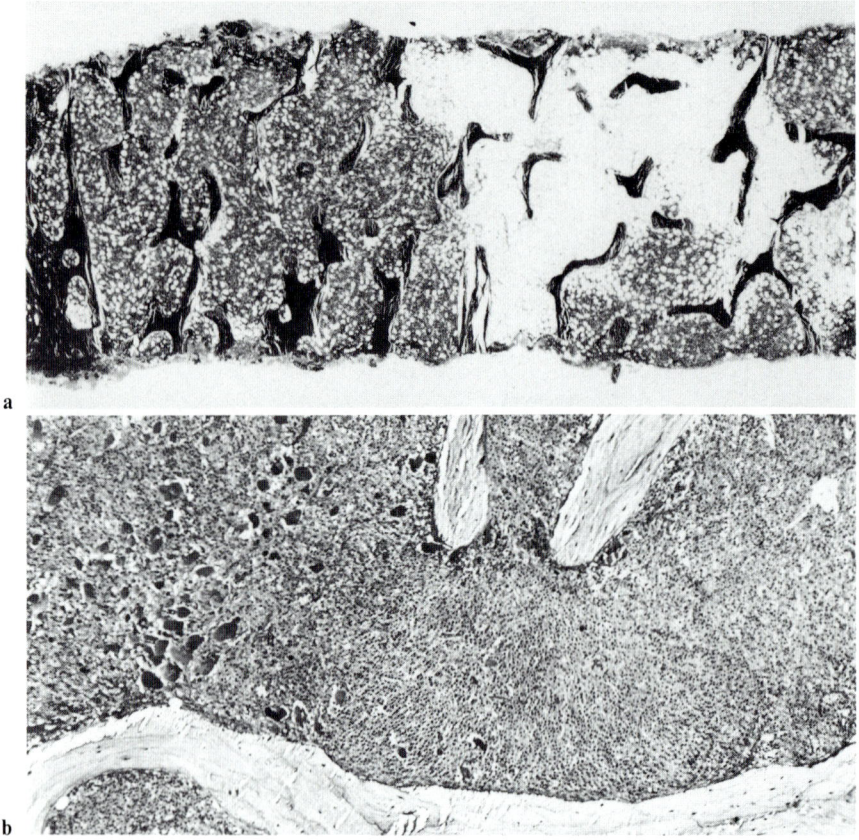

**Fig. 38.** Variations and diagnostic problems of MPD in the bone marrow biopsy. **a** Different patterns of fatty tissue in MegM. Gomori. × 100. **b** Different distribution of megakaryocytes in CML. Giemsa. × 40.

ro-/granulo-/megakaryocytic, (2) erythro-/megakaryocytic, (3) erythro-/granulocytic, and (4) erythrocytic. Transformation of MF/OMS occurs in the two groups with concomitant megakaryocytic proliferation. In MegM two groups are distinguished, the mature and the immature, and both have a high rate of transformation to MF/OMS. In CML, bone marrow histology reveals a granulocytic type, in which metamorphosis to blast crisis frequently occurs, and a mixed, granulo-/megakaryocytic type, in which MF/OMS is likely to supervene.

**Table V.** Histologic classification of MPD

| Clinical entities | Proliferative cell line(s) in the bone marrow | | | Frequency in MPD % | Median survival months[1] | Predominant metamorphosis |
|---|---|---|---|---|---|---|
| PV (191) | ERY | – | – | 3 | 115 | 0 |
| | ERY | GRAN | – | 3 | 99 | 0 |
| | ERY | – | MEG | 27 | 84 | MF/OMS |
| | ERY | GRAN | MEG | 22 | 79 | MF/OMS |
| MegM (53) | – | – | MEG | 14 | 63 | MF/OMS |
| CML (114) | – | GRAN | MEG | 17 | 27 | MF/OMS |
| | – | GRAN | – | 14 | 18 | blast crisis |

[1] Survival time (months) was measured from the time of the biopsy to death or date of last contact.

Our observations demonstrate that the development of MF/OMS in MPD is linked to megakaryocytic proliferation and is thus part of the natural course of the disease. The progressive fibrotic replacement of the original MPD leads to the clinical and histologic entity known as MF/OMS. Patients in this study with myelofibrosis and osteomyelosclerosis had median survivals of about 50 months. For accurate prognostic assessment of patients with MF/OMS, the proliferative disorder should be taken into account: in PV and MegM transformation to MF/OMS indicated a less favourable course, while in CML development of fibrosis decreased the risk of blast crisis.

### References

1   Adamson, J.W.; Fialkow, P.J.: The pathogenesis of myeloproliferative syndromes. Br. J. Haemat. *38:* 299–303 (1978).
2   Bartl, R.; Arzberger, A.; Burkhardt, R.; Fateh-Moghadam, A.: The prognostic significance of the bone marrow histobiopsy in 415 cases of CML. 5th Meet. Int. Soc. Haematol., Afr. Div., Hamburg 1979.
3   Branehög, I.; Ridell, B.; Swolin, B.; Weinfeld, A.: The relation of platelet kinetics to bone marrow megakaryocytes in chronic granulocytic leukaemia. Scand. J. Haematol. *29:* 411–420 (1982).

4   Burkhardt, R.: Bone marrow histology; in Catovsky, Methods in hematology. The leukemic cell, pp. 49–86 (Churchill Livingstone, Edinburgh 1981).

5   Burkhardt, R.; Bartl, R.; Beil, E.; Demmler, K.; Hoffmann, E.; Kronseder, A.; Langegger, H.; Saar, U.; Ulrich, M.; Wiemann, H.: Myelofibrosis-osteosclerosis syndrome. Review of literature and histomorphology; in Advances in the bio-sciences, vol. 16, pp. 9–56 (Pergamon Press, Oxford/Vieweg, Braunschweig 1975).

6   Burkhardt, R.; Bartl, R.: Histobioptische Differentialdiagnose und Prognose der myeloproliferativen Störungen; in Wilmanns, Hartenstein, Beitr. Onkol., vol. 13, pp. 201–224 (Karger, Basel 1982).

7   Burkhardt, R.; Frisch, B.; Bartl, R.: Bone biopsy in haematological disorders. J. clin. Path. *35:* 257–284 (1982).

8   Burkhardt, R.; Cirl, C.; Bartl, R.; Jäger, K.: 193 histobioptic case controls in 58 polycythaemic patients in the course of 2–15 years. 5th Meet. Int. Soc. Haematol., Eur. Afr. Div., Hamburg 1979.

9   Caligaris Cappio, F.; Vigliani, R.; Novariono, A.; Camussi, G.; Campana, D.; Gavos-to, F.: Idiopathic myelofibrosis: a possible role for immune-complexes in the patho-genesis of bone marrow fibrosis. Br. J. Haemat. *49:* 17–21 (1981).

10  Castro-Malaspina, H.; Moore, M.A.S.: Pathophysiological mechanisms operating in the development of myelofibrosis: role of megakaryocytes. Nouv. Revue fr. Hémat. *24:* 221–226 (1982).

11  Clough, V.; Geary, C.G.; Hashmi, K.; Knowlson, T.: Myelofibrosis in chronic gran-ulocytic leukemia. Br. J. Haemat. *42:* 515–526 (1979).

12  Dameshek, W.: Myeloproliferative disorders. Blood *6:* 372–375 (1951).

13  Ellis, J.T.; Silver, R.T.; Coleman, M.; Celler, S.A.: The bone marrow in polycythemia vera. Semin. Hematol. *12:* 433–444 (1975).

14  Fialkow, P.J.; Faguet, G.B.; Jacobson, R.J.; Vaidya, K.; Murphy, S.: Evidence that essential thrombocythemia is a clonal disorder with origin in a multipotent stem cell. Blood *58:* 916–919 (1982).

15  Frisch, B.; Bartl, R.; Burkhardt, R.: Bone marrow biopsy in clinical medicine: an overview. Haematologia *3:* 245–285 (1982).

16  Georgii, A.: Histopathology of bone marrow in human chronic leukemias; in Neth, Galco, Hofschneider, Mannweiler, Modern trends in human leukemia, vol. II, pp. 59–70 (Springer, Berlin 1975).

17  Georgii, A.: Klassifikation der chronischen myeloproliferativen Erkrankungen durch Histopathologie und Zytogenetik des Knochenmarkes; in Wilmanns, Hartenstein, Beitr. Onkol., vol. 13, pp. 166–188 (Karger, Basel 1982).

18  Georgii, A.; Thiele, J.; Vykoupil, K.F.: Osteomyelofibrosis/-sclerosis: a histological and cytogenetic study on core biopsies of the bone marrow. Virchows Arch. Abt. A Path. Anat. *389:* 269–286 (1980).

19  Gilbert, H.S.: The spectrum of myeloproliferative disorders; in Rubin, Clinical signs of blood disease. The medical clinics of North America, vol. 57/2, pp. 355–393 (Saunders, Philadelphia 1973).

20  Gordon, B.R.; Coleman, M.; Kohen, P.; Day, N.K.: Immunologic abnormalities in myelofibrosis with activation of the complement system. Blood *58:* 904–910 (1981).

21  Groopman, J.E.: The pathogenesis of myelofibrosis in myeloproliferative disorders. Ann. intern. Med. *92:* 857–858 (1980).

22  Jacobson, R.J.; Salo, A.; Fialkow, P.J.: Agnogenic myeloid metaplasia: a clonal pro-
    liferation of hematopoietic stem cells with secondary myelofibrosis. Blood *51:* 189–
    194 (1978).
23  Jamshidi, K.; Ansari, A.; Windschitl, H.E.; Swaim, W.R.: Primary thrombocythe-
    mia. Geriatrics *28:* 121 (1973).
24  Koeffler, H.P.; Golde, D.W.: Chronic myelogenous leukemia: new concepts. New
    Engl. J. Med. *304:* 1201–1209 (1981).
25  Laszlo, J.: Myeloproliferative disorders (MPD): myelofibrosis, myelosclerosis, extra-
    medullary hematopoiesis, undifferentiated MPD, and hemorrhagic thrombocythe-
    mia. Semin. Hematol. *12:* 409–432 (1975).
26  Lundin, P.M.; Ridell, B.; Weinfeld, A.: The significance of bone marrow morphol-
    ogy for the diagnosis of polycythemia vera. Scand. J. Haematol. *9:* 271–282 (1977).
27  Manoharan, A.; Smart, R.C.; Pitney, W.R.: Prognostic factors in myelofibrosis.
    Pathology *14:* 455–461 (1982).
28  McGlave, P.B.; Brunning, R.D.; Hurdand, D.D.; Kim, T.H.: Reversal of severe bone
    marrow fibrosis and osteosclerosis following allogeneic bone marrow transplantation
    for chronic granulocytic leukaemia. Br. J. Haemat. *52:* 189–194 (1982).
29  Moore, M.A.S.: Pathogenesis of MF; in Hoffbrand, Recent advances in haematology,
    pp. 136–139 (Churchill Livingstone, Edinburgh 1982).
30  Murphy, S.: Thrombocytosis and thrombocythaemia. Clin. Haematol. *12:* 89–106
    (1983).
31  Nowell, P.C.; Hungerford, D.A.: A minute chromosome in human chronic granulo-
    cytic leukemia. Science *132:* 1497 (1960).
32  Pettit, J.E.: The non-leukaemic myeloproliferative disorders; in Hoffbrand, Lewis,
    Postgraduate haematology, 2nd ed., pp. 577–604 (Heinemann, London 1981).
33  Prechtel, K.; Beil, E.; Kronseder, A.: Megakaryozytäre Myelose, Klinik und Morpho-
    logie. Dt. med. Wschr. *102:* 853 (1977).
34  Ross, R.; Vogel, A.: The platelet-derived growth factor. Cell *14:* 203–210 (1978).
35  Spiers, A.S.D.: Metamorphosis of chronic granulocytic leukaemia: diagnosis, classifi-
    cation and management. Br. J. Haemat. *41:* 1–7 (1979).
36  Strebel, U.; Schaffner, A.; Fehr, J.: Die akute Osteomyelofibrose. Schweiz. med.
    Wschr. *113:* 844–850 (1983).
37  Thiele, J.; Holgado, S.; Choritz, H.; Georgii, A.: Density distribution and size of
    megakaryocytes in inflammatory reactions of the bone marrow (myelitis) and chronic
    myeloproliferative diseases. Scand. J. Haematol. *31:* 329–341 (1983).

# 5 Adult Acute Leukaemias (AL)

**Survey of the Literature**

Reports in the literature deal almost exclusively with cytologic and cytochemical investigations [1–3, 6, 8, 14, 17, 20, 22]. Initially the only prognostically relevant factor to emerge was the distinction between myeloid and lymphoid leukaemias. In the past decade most investigations carried out to identify factors of prognostic significance have employed enzymic characteristics and immunologic markers [4, 6, 10, 13, 23, 24]. However, their prognostic relevance is not yet established so that the initial white cell count and the morphologic features, on which the French-American-British (FAB) classification is based, still provide the most reliable indicators of prognosis [1, 5]. These have been extensively reviewed recently [4, 25]. In contrast, studies on bone marrow histology in the acute leukaemias have been few and far between [7, 12, 18, 19]. One structural characteristic which has received attention is the reticulin fibre content in the leukaemic infiltrations. *Kundel* et al. [15] stated that acute leukaemias with an increase in reticulin fibres in the bone marrow did not respond well to chemotherapy and had a poorer life expectancy. Similarly, *Manoharan* et al. [16] noted that reticulin fibres decreased when the leukaemia was successfully treated and reappeared with the occurrence of relapse. They offered no explanation to account for this association. Likewise, only a few data are available on the prognostic value of other histologic criteria such as the proliferation patterns and the volume percentages of infiltration, haematopoiesis and fat in the bone marrow biopsy [12, 14].

If one summarizes reports in the literature, it appears that the cytologic and cytochemical classifications in use are not entirely satisfactory with respect to prediction of the effects of therapy [5, 9], while the more sophisticated techniques such as cytogenetic analysis, quantitative cytochemistry, proliferation kinetics and immunologic surface markers have yet to prove their values as reliable prognostic indicators in large series of patients [4, 10, 11, 23].

### Own Observations

We investigated 205 bone marrow biopsies of 182 adult patients with AL. In each case the first biopsy was performed for initial diagnosis before specific therapeutic regimens were instituted. In this retrospective study the patients were cared for in various hospitals and haematologic centres and consequently received different treatment regimens. Though our survival data are not comparable with the results of more recent prospective studies, the prognostic assessment of various histologic parameters in AL may be informative with respect to further prospective studies. The initial diagnosis of AL was based on established cytologic (FAB system), cytochemical and clinical criteria. The marrows smears or imprints of the biopsies were stained with May-Grünwald-Giemsa, PAS, peroxidase and, if required, alpha-naphthylacetate esterase. Survival data were available for all the 169 patients registered. 9 histologic parameters were analyzed for their prognostic relevance in AL.

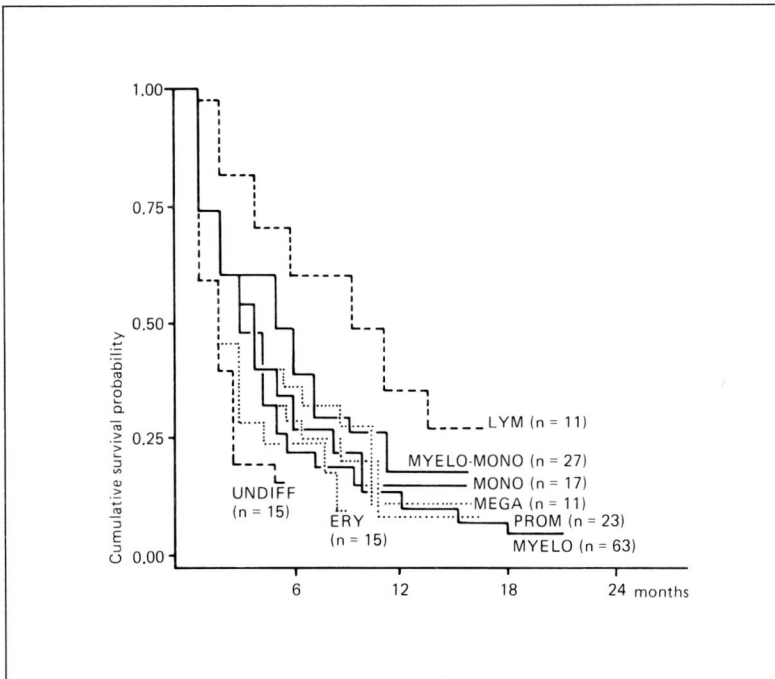

**Fig. 39.** Predictive value of bone marrow histology in AL; grouping variable is 'proliferative cell type'.

**Table VI.** Prognostic factors of AL in the bone marrow biopsy

| Histologic criteria | Patients | Median survival months | Breslow, Mantel-Cox p values |
|---|---|---|---|
| Proliferative cell type | | | 0.1262 |
| Undifferentiated | 15 | 2 | 0.1672 |
| Lymphoblastic | 11 | 10 | |
| Myeloblastic | 63 | 3 | |
| Myelomonocytic | 27 | 5 | |
| Monoblastic | 17 | 3 | |
| Promyelocytic | 23 | 3 | |
| Erythroblastic | 15 | 2 | |
| Megakaryoblastic | 11 | 4 | |
| Fatty tissue | | | 0.0803 |
| < 20 vol% | 140 | 3 | 0.0412 |
| ≥ 20 vol% | 28 | 10 | |
| Fibrosis | | | 0.1022 |
| Fine | 144 | 4 | 0.0620 |
| Coarse | 25 | 2 | |

*Identification of Prognostic Factors in*
*Bone Marrow Histology*

Grouping according to the proliferative cell type demonstrated that adult patients with lymphoblastic leukaemia had a more favourable course than those with non-lymphoblastic leukaemias (fig. 39, table VI). The rare forms of AL with concomitant myelodysplastic features – the promyelocytic, erythroblastic and megakaryoblastic types – also showed an unfavourable prognosis (fig. 39). Two histologic variables had predictive value, in addition to the cytologic cell type: the content of fat cells and the degree of fibrosis. Patients with a high content of fat cells, diffusely dispersed among the leukaemic blasts (interstitial pattern), had longer survival times than those without fat cells (packed marrow pattern) (fig. 40, table VI). This correlation was also found in myeloblastic leukaemia, the largest group of AL

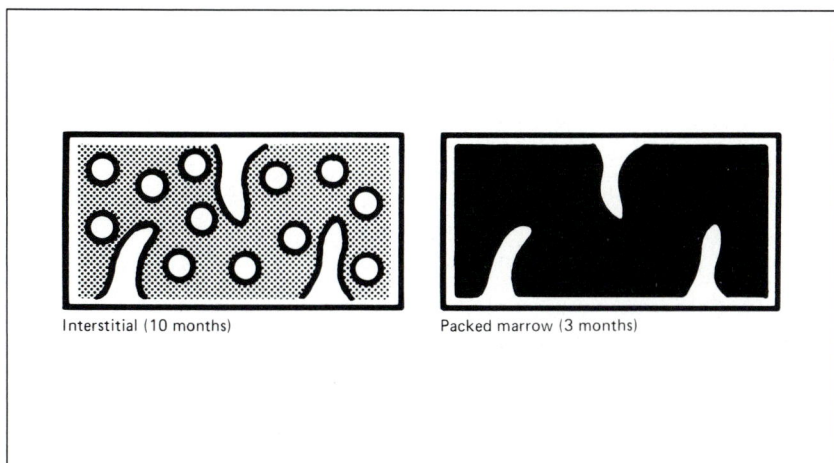

Interstitial (10 months)              Packed marrow (3 months)

**Fig. 40.** Patterns of AL in the bone marrow histology and their prognostic relevance (median survival time).

(fig. 41, 42). An increase in reticulin fibres indicated shorter survival times (table VI). Mitotic activity was not an independent factor, as it was linked to the morphologic cell type. The content of siderin and of plasma cells in the marrow had no significant influence on prognosis.

*Histologic Classification*

Morphologic classification of AL was made by both bone marrow histology and smears of imprints (table VII). There was complete agreement between the results of these techniques in 80% of the cases (excluding the promyelocytic, erythroblastic and megakaryoblastic types). In another 15% of the cases cytochemistry established the diagnosis of the leukaemic cell type. 5% could not be classified by morphology or cytochemistry: these were called the 'undifferentiated' type. The AL with myelodysplastic features, i.e. the promyelocytic, erythroblastic and megakaryoblastic leukaemias, were more reliably diagnosed by histology which revealed a characteristic histotopographic arrangement in the bone marrow. The histologic features of the different types of AL are illustrated in figures 43 and 44, the survival curves of the patients are shown in figure 39.

**Table VII.** Histologic classification of AL – 182 untreated patients at time of initial biopsy

|  | Undifferentiated | Lymphoblastic | Myeloblastic | Myelomonocytic | Monoblastic | Promyelocytic | Erythroblastic | Megakaryoblastic |
|---|---|---|---|---|---|---|---|---|
| Patients | 15 | 11 | 63 | 27 | 17 | 23 | 15 | 11 |
| Male/female | 1.5 | 1.6 | 0.4 | 0.5 | 0.3 | 2.7 | 1.3 | 2.5 |
| Age, median, years | 56 | 31 | 51 | 46 | 55 | 71 | 59 | 62 |
| Lymphomas, % | 60 | 42 | 25 | 28 | 45 | 16 | 13 | 15 |
| Splenomegaly, % | 40 | 55 | 48 | 52 | 60 | 25 | 50 | 32 |
| Hepatomegaly, % | 60 | 50 | 42 | 45 | 45 | 43 | 60 | 58 |
| Anaemia (Hb <8 g/dl), % | 40 | 30 | 25 | 32 | 30 | 25 | 50 | 25 |
| Leukopenia (<4 × $10^9$/l), % | 40 | 20 | 10 | 40 | 22 | 32 | 53 | 50 |
| Leukocytosis (>10 × $10^9$/l), % | 40 | 50 | 44 | 50 | 44 | 20 | 20 | 35 |
| Thrombopenia (<100 × $10^9$/l), % | 80 | 55 | 73 | 70 | 89 | 78 | 78 | 45 |
| Leukaemic blood picture, % | 60 | 60 | 50 | 70 | 55 | 40 | 20 | 50 |
| Infiltration, vol% | 60 (20) | 60 (21) | 51 (25) | 60 (15) | 65 (18) | 40 (31) | 36 (10) | 32 (21) |
| Infiltration, <20 vol%, % | 0 | 8 | 16 | 0 | 9 | 25 | 40 | 44 |
| Haematopoietic tissue, vol% | 4 (4) | 4 (6) | 10 (21) | 6 (6) | 6 (10) | 23 (25) | 26 (10) | 30 (12) |
| Fatty tissue, vol% | 8 (10) | 6 (6) | 10 (10) | 8 (11) | 4 (3) | 6 (5) | 5 (7) | 5 (6) |
| Sinusoids, vol% | 3 (5) | 1 (1) | 2 (2) | 2 (2) | 1 (1) | 3 (2) | 4 (3) | 3 (2) |
| Trabecular bone, vol% | 21 (4) | 24 (6) | 22 (4) | 23 (4) | 21 (4) | 22 (4) | 21 (4) | 22 (4) |
| Lymphoid nodules, % | 0 | 0 | 5 | 0 | 0 | 4 | 8 | 9 |

Numbers in parentheses = standard deviations.

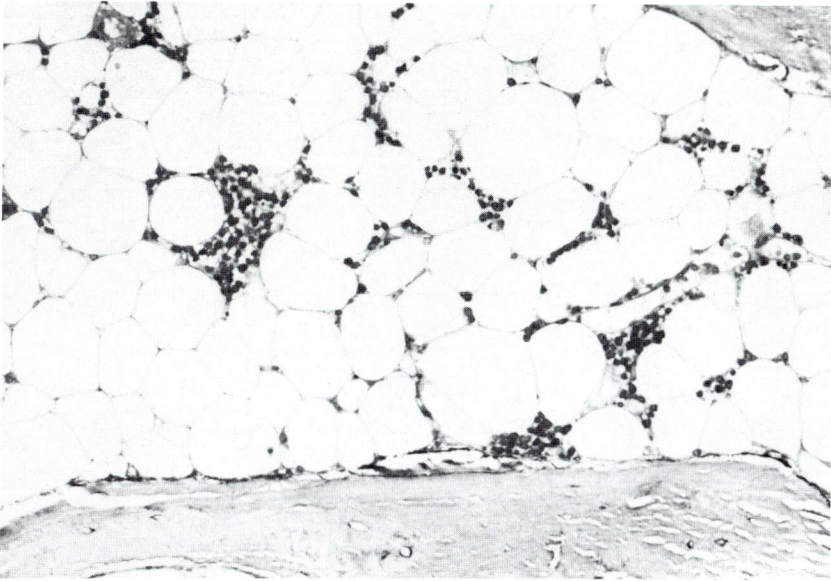

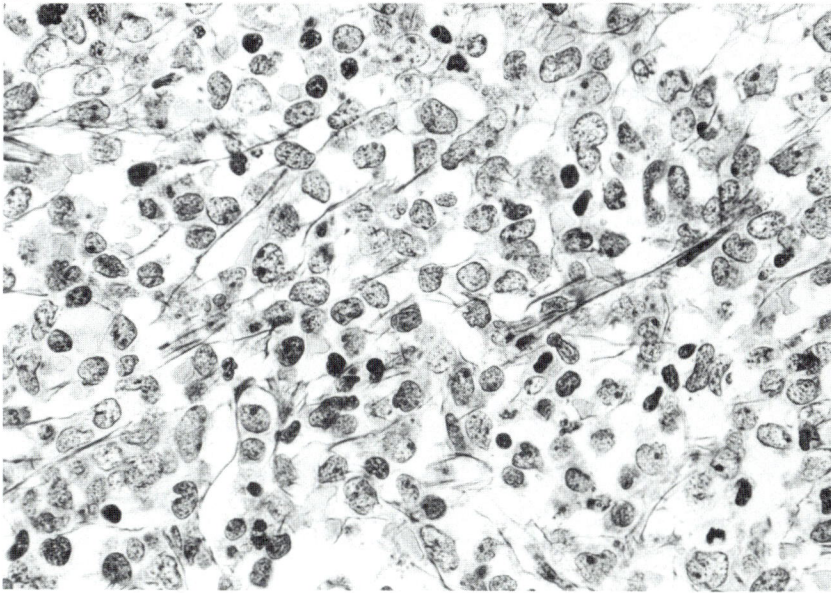

**Fig. 41.** Hypocellular type of myeloblastic leukaemia with loose distribution of myeloblasts between the fat cells. Complete lack of normal haematopoiesis. Giemsa. × 100.

**Fig. 42.** Coarse fibrosis in myeloblastic leukaemia. Gomori. × 400.

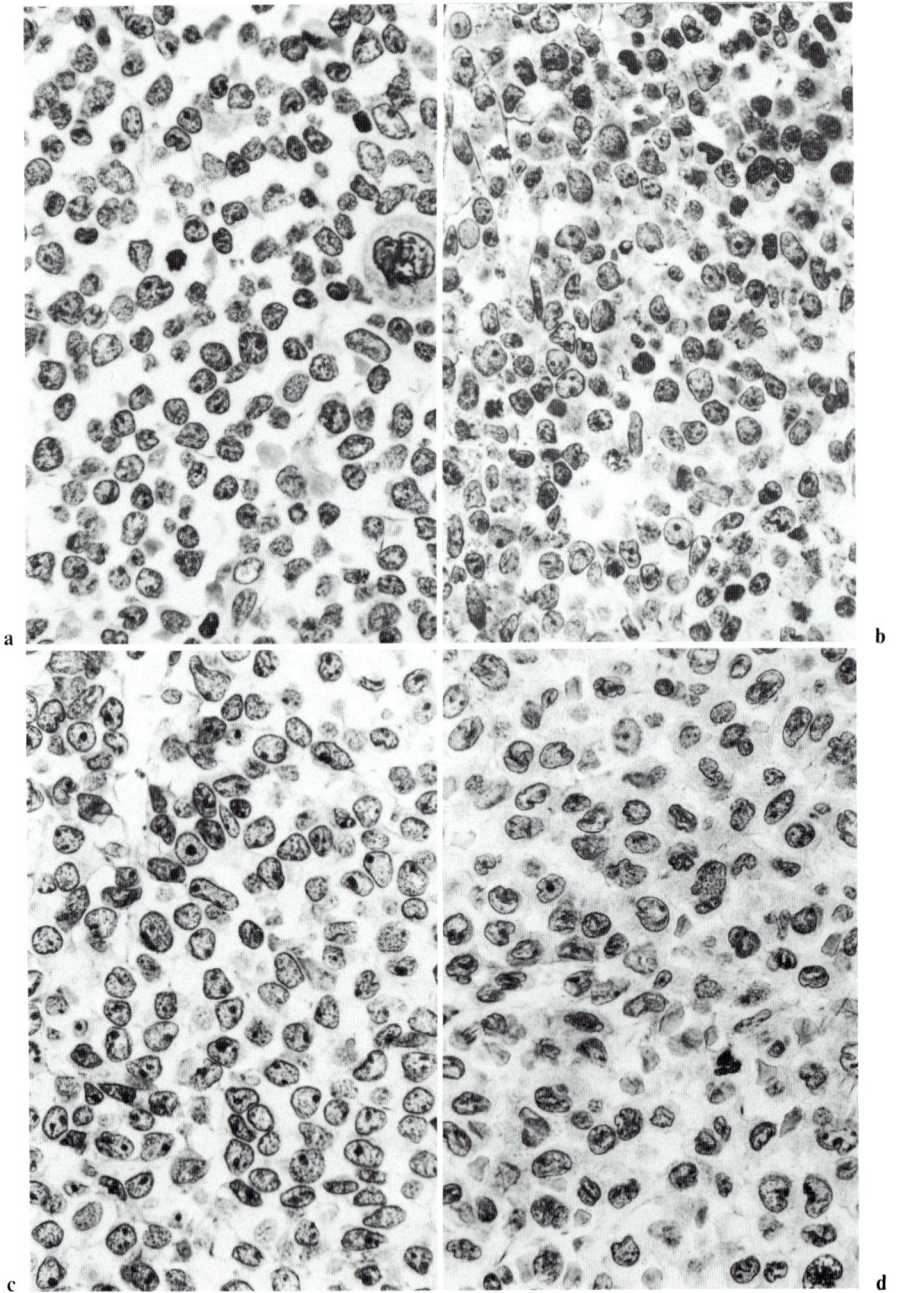

**Fig. 43.** Legend p. 54.

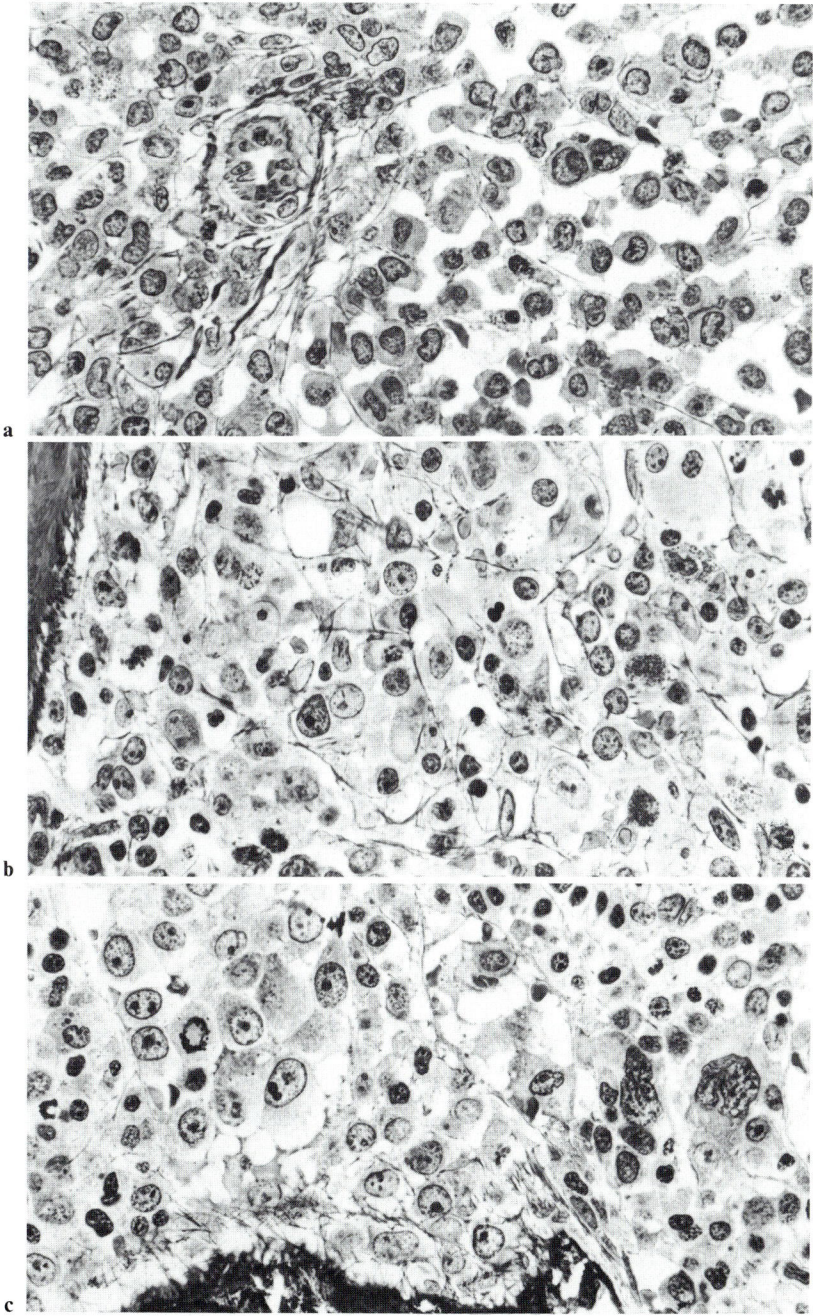

**Fig. 44.** Legend p. 54.

## Implications for Medical Practice

Smears of peripheral blood or bone marrow aspirates are routinely used for diagnosis and classification of AL. Bone marrow biopsy is usually performed only because of a dry tap [19]. With increasing understanding of the role of the haematopoietic microenvironment and other stromal elements, bone marrow biopsies in AL as well as in preleukaemia (fig. 45) will undoubtedly be reported more frequently. We have shown that the quantitative estimation of the leukaemic infiltration in the bone marrow had predictive value. AL patients with interstitial patterns had a relatively indolent course of disease and corresponded to the clinical group of 'smouldering leukaemias'. However, marked variations of blastic infiltration in different areas of the same biopsy (fig. 46) must be considered. Furthermore, demonstration of coarse fibrosis indicated an unfavourable prognosis. An increase in the reticulin fibre content in the bone marrow of patients in remission is thought to be associated with relapse [16]. In AL with myelodysplastic features, i.e. the promyelocytic, erythroblastic (di Guglielmo) and megakaryoblastic types, the bone marrow biopsy proved to be a prerequisite for diagnosis because of the high incidence of dry taps and the diagnostic value of the histotopographic growth patterns revealed in the biopsy section. Furthermore, bone marrow biopsy may be a more effective way to check induction of complete remission in AL and to monitor the effects of therapy, than examination of peripheral blood or aspirates alone.

**Fig. 43.** Histologic types of AL in the bone marrow. Gomori. × 250. **a** AL lymphoblastic. **b** AL myeloblastic. **c** AL myelomonocytic. **d** AL monoblastic. Verification of the histologic diagnosis by cytology and cytochemistry.

**Fig. 44.** Histologic types of AL (with myelodysplastic features) in the bone marrow. Gomori. × 250. **a** AL promyelocytic. **b** AL erythroblastic. **c** AL megakaryoblastic.

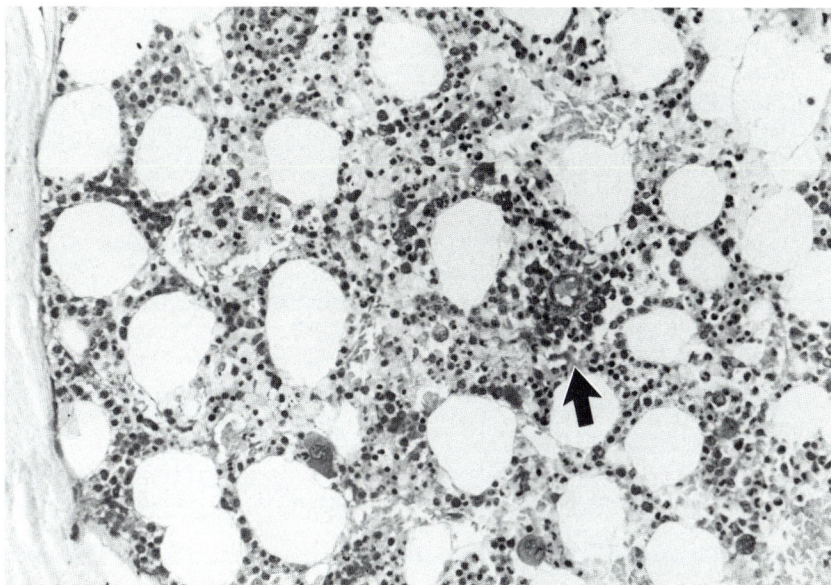

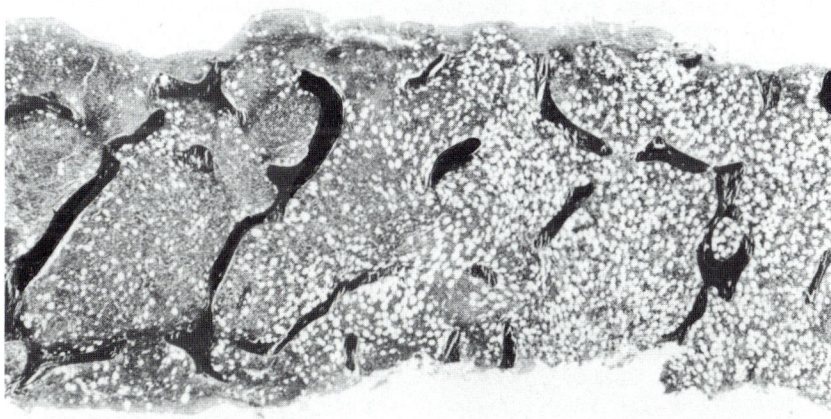

**Fig. 45.** Preleukaemia with marked exsudative reaction of the stroma, extravasates of erythrocytes and myelodysplastic changes. Precursors of granulopoiesis in the perivascular region (arrow). Giemsa. × 100. Two months later, the sequential biopsy revealed the typical features of myeloblastic leukaemia.

**Fig. 46.** Variation of blastic infiltration in lymphoblastic leukaemia. Gomori. × 10.

## References

1   Aul, C.; Fischer, J.T.; Schneider, W.: Zytologisch-zytochemische Methoden in der Klassifikation akuter Leukämien. Dt. med. Wschr. *16:* 631–638 (1983).

2   Bennet, J.M.; Catovsky, D.; Daniel, M.T.; Flandrin, G.; Galton, D.A.G.; Gralnick, H.R.; Sultan, C.: Proposals for the classification of the acute leukaemias. Br. J. Haemat. *33:* 451 (1976).

3   Catovsky, D.: The leukemic cell (Churchill Livingstone, Edinburgh 1981).

4   Catovsky, D.; Tavares de Castro, J.: The classification of acute leukaemia (AL) and its clinical significance. Schweiz. med. Wschr. *113:* 1434–1437 (1983).

5   Cavalli, P.: Prognostische Faktoren und Therapie der akuten Leukämien beim Erwachsenen (Huber, Bern 1980).

6   Creutzig, U.; Schellong, G.: Differenzierung der akuten Leukämien. Dt. med. Wschr. *40:* 1303–1308 (1981).

7   Demmler, K.; Burkhardt, R.; Prechtel, K.: Megakaryoblastische Myelose. Klin. Wschr. *48:* 1168–1173 (1970).

8   Flandrin, G.; Bernard, J.: Cytological classification of acute leukemias. A survey of 1,400 cases; in Bessis, Brecher, Unclassifiable leukaemias, pp. 7–15 (Springer, Berlin 1975).

9   Foon, K.A.; Naiem, F.; Yale, C.; Gale, R.P.: Acute myelogenous leukemia: morphologic classification and response to therapy. Leuk. Res. *3:* 171–173 (1979).

10  Gordon, D.S.; Hubbar, M.: Surface membrane characteristics and cytochemistry of the abnormal cells in adult acute leukemia. Blood *51:* 681–692 (1978).

11  Hart, J.S.; George, S.L.; Frei, E.; Bodey, G.P.; Nickerson, R.C.; Freireich, E.J.: Prognostic significance of pretreatment proliferative activity in adult acute leukemia. Cancer *39:* 1603–1617 (1977).

12  Howe, R.B.; Bloomfield, C.D.; McKenna, R.W.: Hypocellular acute leukemia. Am. J. Med. *72:* 391–395 (1982).

13  Janossy, G.; Hoffbrand, A.V.; Greaves, M.F.; Ganeshaguru, K.; Pain, C.; Bradstock, K.F.; Prentice, H.G.; Kay, H.E.M.; Lister, T.A.: Terminal transferase enzyme assay and immunological membrane markers in the diagnosis of leukaemia: a multiparameter analysis of 300 cases. Br. J. Haemat. *44:* 221–234 (1980).

14  Keating, M.J.; Smith, T.L.; Gehan, E.A.; McCredie, K.B.; Bodey, G.P.; Freireich, E.J.: A prognostic factor analysis for use in development of predictive models for response in adult acute leukemia. Cancer *50:* 457–465 (1982).

15  Kundel, D.W.; Brecher, G.; Bodey, G.P.; Brittin, G.M.: Reticulin fibrosis and bone infarction in acute leukemia. Implications for prognosis. Blood *23:* 526–544 (1964).

16  Manoharan, D.; Horsley, R.; Pitney, W.R.: The reticulin content of bone marrow in acute leukaemia in adults. Br. J. Haemat. *43:* 185–190 (1979).

17  Mirchandani, I.; Palutke, M.: Acute megakaryoblastic leukemia. Cancer *50:* 2866–2872 (1983).

18  Ottolander, G.J.; Velde, J. te; Bredow, P.; Geraerdt, J.P.M.; Slee, P.H.T.; Willemze, R.; Zwaan, F.E.; Haak, H.L.; Muller, H.P.; Bieger, R.: Megakaryoblastic leukaemia (acute myelofibrosis). Br. J. Haemat. *42:* 9–20 (1979).

19  Rappaport, H.: Histologic criteria for diagnosis and classification of acute leukemias; in Mathé, Puillart, Schwarzenberg, Nomenclature, methodology and results of clinical trials in acute leukemias, pp. 35–42 (Springer, Berlin 1973).

20  Medical Research Council's Working Party on Leukaemia in Adults: The relation between morphology and other features of acute myeloid leukaemia, and their prognostic significance. Br. J. Haemat. *31:* 165–180 (1975).
21  Shaw, M.T.: The cytochemistry of acute leukemia: a diagnostic and prognostic evaluation. Semin. Oncol. *3:* 219–228 (1976).
22  Slyck van, E.J.; Rebuck, J.W.; Waddell, C.C.; Janakiraman, N.: Smoldering acute granulocytic leukemia. Archs intern. Med. *143:* 37–40 (1983).
23  Thiel, E.: Monoclonal antibodies against differentiation antigens of lymphopoiesis. Blut *47:* 247–261 (1983).
24  Thierfelder, S.; Rodt, H.; Thiel, E.; Hoffmann-Fezer, G.; Netzel, H.; Haas, R.J.; Wündisch, G.F.; Bender-Götze, C.: Immunologic markers for classification of leukemias and non-Hodgkin lymphomas; in Gross, Hellriegel, Recent results in cancer research, vol. 69: Strategies in clinical hematology, pp. 41–48 (Springer, Berlin 1979).
25  Whittaker, J.A.; Withey, J.; Powell, D.E.B.; Parry, T.E.; Kurshid, M.: Leukaemia classification: a study of the accuracy of diagnosis in 456 patients. Br. J. Haemat. *41:* 177–184 (1979).

# 6   Multiple Myeloma (MM)

## Survey of the Literature

Normal plasma cells are derived from B lymphocytes by transformation (fig. 6), and each plasma cell produces only one type of immunoglobulin. In myeloma all the malignant cells secrete the same immunoglobulin indicating that they arose by proliferation of a single cell: the disease is therefore monoclonal [13, 20]. Furthermore, it appears that most plasma cell neoplasias are stem cell disorders [23, 27, 32]. When a plasma cell clone has expanded to a size of $10^{10}$, it may be detectable as a gammapathy due to the secretion of a globulin into the plasma. Such a clone may involute, persist or progress to malignant transformation, the MM. $10^{11}$ to $10^{12}$ cells, corresponding to a tumour weight of 100–1,000 g, are required for MM to become clinically evident [14, 30]. The progression of MM is extremely variable, it has a long preclinical stage, a variable symptomatic stage and may have a smouldering course of up to 14 years [10, 19, 22]. MM is the only type of B-neoplasm which is primarily localized to the bone marrow. It stimulates osteoclastic activity which in turn produces lytic lesions in the skeleton [15, 33]. Thus the classic trilogy diagnostic of MM is established: a monoclonal immunoglobulin in the plasma, osteolytic lesions on X ray and a plasmacytosis of more than 30% in smears of bone marrow aspirates [16, 21, 25, 29, 31]. Three types of plasma cell neoplasias have been distinguished on the basis of tumour growth patterns: (1) multiple myeloma, systemic from the outset and comprising more than 90% of the plasma cell neoplasias [2, 4], (2) plasma cell sarcoma, characterized by a metastatic behaviour [12], and (3) solitary plasmacytoma, within the skeleton or in extraosseous sites and characterized by adenomatous growth [7].

Numerous authors have commented on the close association between the morphologic picture of MM and its prognosis. As early as 1948 – that is before the introduction of cytostatic therapy – *Bayrd* [8] drew attention to the fact that the degree of differentiation of the myeloma cells affected the survival duration of the patients. Without therapy, patients with mature-type plasma cells had a life expectancy of up to 6 years, while those with immature cells died within a year. In 1954, *Astaldi* et al. [3] observed that the cells of an 'immature' plasmacytoma had a faster rate of proliferation and a less favourable prognosis. These observations were later confirmed by others [31]. *Kyle and Bayrd* [20] studied a large series of myeloma patients to determine prognostic factors and found that those with differentiated myeloma cells had longer survivals. *Beer* et al. [9] as well as *Kiang* et al. [18] also noted the connection between cellular morphology and duration of survival. In 1973, *Azar and Potter* [4] proposed a grading system in which they subdivided the myeloma cells into three grades according to the degree of differentiation, but statistical confirmation of its prognostic relevance was not provided. *Kapadia* [17], using a histologic grading system, divided 62 autopsy cases of MM into three groups. When correlated with the extent of disease on gross examination, he found that approximately 80% of cases with grade 1 and 66% with grade 2 myeloma cells had stage I disease. Patients with grade 3 myeloma cells usually had stage II disease at autopsy. However, he found no correlation between the type of M component, treatment or survival with the stage of disease or the histologic grade of the myeloma cells. On the other hand, *Vercelli* et al. [34, 35] reported a close relationship between the percentage of myeloma cells in smears of aspirates and survival. *Kyle and Greipp* [22] observed 6 patients with smouldering MM who had only a moderate plasmacytosis in smears of aspirates.

## Own Observations

A total of 245 patients with MM was investigated. Diagnosis of MM was based on the clinical criteria employed by the Southwest Oncology Group [13]. Of the 16 doubtful cases, 10 were identified unequivocally as MM by immunohistologic methods performed on cryostat sections of the bone marrow (technique described in chapter 2). Furthermore the initial diagnosis of all patients were verified in follow-up studies. Once the initial diagnosis of all patients was made, and after the first biopsy, therapy with melphalan and prednisone was instituted according to the clinical requirements. In 220 (90%) of the 245 patients with MM bone marrow manifestation was found in the biopsy. Survival data were available for all MM patients included in this report. Sequential biopsies were obtained in 64 patients. The remaining 10% of MM patients with negative initial biopsies revealed bone marrow involvement in sequential biopsies, performed to evaluate the effects of therapy.

### *Identification of Prognostic Factors in Bone Marrow Histology*

14 histologic parameters were assessed to determine their predictive value. The most significant prognostic factor proved to be the maturity of the plasma cells (table VIII). The plasma cells were initially grouped into

**Table VIII.** Prognostic factors of MM in the bone marrow biopsy

| Histologic criteria | Patients | Median survival months | Breslow, Mantel-Cox p values |
|---|---|---|---|
| Cell maturity |  |  | 0.0001 |
| Mature | 149 | 32 | 0.0002 |
| Immature | 71 | 8 |  |
| Growth pattern |  |  | 0.0009 |
| Interstitial | 79 | 35 | 0.0006 |
| Myelomatous | 97 | 18 |  |
| Packed marrow | 44 | 9 |  |
| Infiltration |  |  | 0.0025 |
| < 20 vol% | 72 | 128 | 0.0012 |
| 20–50 vol% | 102 | 18 |  |
| > 50 vol% | 46 | 10 |  |
| Fibrosis |  |  | 0.0003 |
| Fine | 165 | 42 | 0.0002 |
| Coarse | 55 | 16 |  |

three grades of maturity – mature, intermediate and immature – for which the presence of nucleoli was the most important parameter. When the survival data were computed, significant differences were found only between the curves for the mature group and the two others together (median survivals of 32, 8 and 7 months, respectively). Therefore, from a prognostic point of view, only two histologic grades were subsequently distinguished: mature and immature (fig. 47). Highly significant differences were found in the survival test statistics of these two groups (table VIII). Additional cytologic criteria with significant predictive value proved to be the degree of plasma cell atypia and the mitotic activity. Polymorphous plasma cells and a high mitotic activity indicated an unfavourable prognosis. Of the histomorphometric variables the volume percentages of plasma cell infiltration and of fat cells in the biopsy showed significant prognostic value (table VIII). A high plasma cell burden as well as a low proportion of fatty tissue correlated with shorter survival times (fig. 48). The patients were also categorized according to the proliferation pattern in the biopsy: interstitial, interstitial with 'myelomas' (myelomatous), and packed marrow (fig. 49).

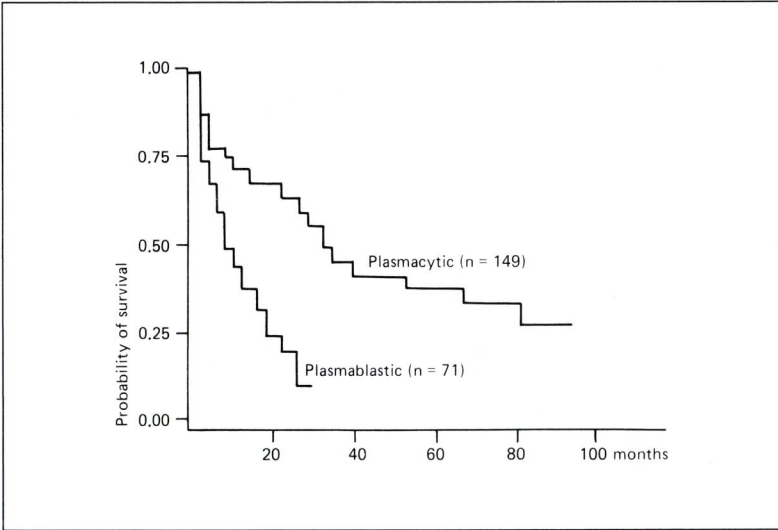

**Fig. 47.** Predictive value of bone marrow histology in MM; grouping variable is 'plasma cell maturity'.

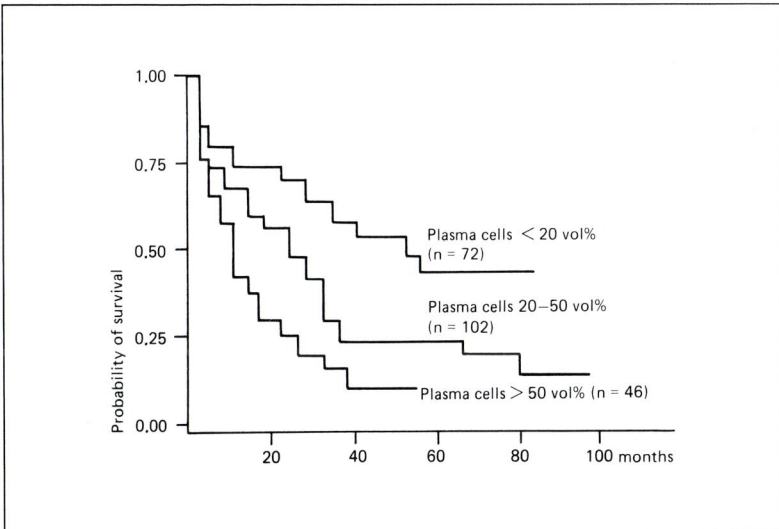

**Fig. 48.** Predictive value of bone marrow histology in MM; grouping variable is 'infiltration volume in the biopsy (vol%)'.

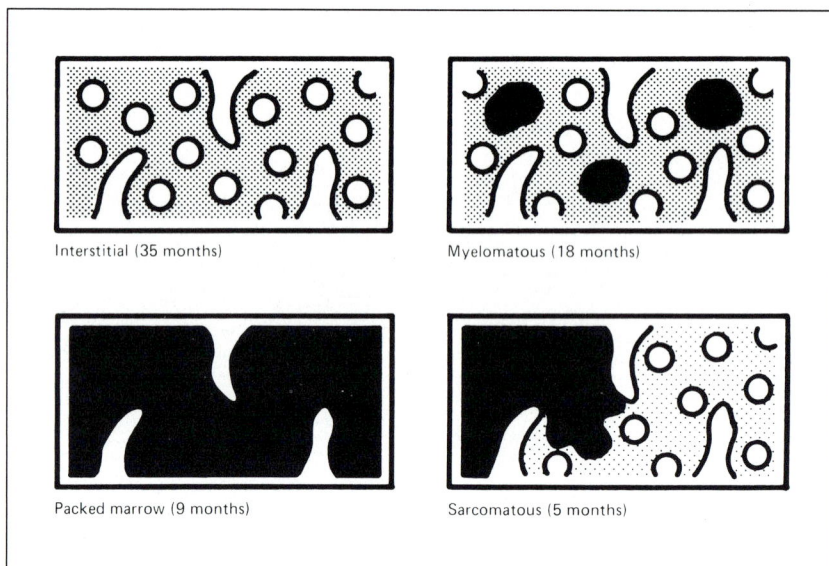

Fig. 49. Patterns of MM in the bone marrow histology and their prognostic relevance (median survival time).

Those with an interstitial bone marrow pattern had the longest, and those with a packed marrow pattern had the shortest median survival times (table VIII). Non-specific changes, such as fibrosis, bone remodelling and trabecular bone volume also proved to be useful in predicting survival duration, with p values lower than 0.01 in the Mantel-Cox test (table VIII). The presence of siderin and of small lymphoid nodules correlated with longer survivals, though not significantly.

*Histologic Classification*

Because of their prognostic significance and the advantage of their reproducibility, the histologic criteria of cellular maturity and infiltration volume percentage were further analyzed to test their suitability for classification and staging of MM (table IX). For this purpose the biopsies were divided into two categories: plasmacytic and plasmablastic. The *plasmacytic type* was characterized by typical, differentiated plasma cells, though there were variations in size, with a spectrum of 'micro' plasma cells resembling lymphocytes to 'hypertrophied' plasma cells with abundant cytoplasm (fig. 50a). Mitotic activity was not observed. The growth pattern was inter-

**Table IX.** Histologic classification of MM – 220 untreated patients at time of initial biopsy

|  | Plasmacytic | Plasmablastic |
|---|---|---|
| Patients | 149 | 71 |
| Male/female | 0.9 | 1.4 |
| Age, median, years | 66 | 55 |
| Osteoporosis (X ray), % | 25 | 26 |
| Osteolysis (X ray), % | 42 | 33 |
| Osteosclerosis (X ray), % | 3 | 1 |
| Splenomegaly, % | 9 | 17 |
| Hepatomegaly, % | 27 | 37 |
| Anaemia (Hb < 10 g/dl), % | 22 | 49 |
| Leukopenia (< 4 × 10$^9$/l), % | 12 | 10 |
| Thrombopenia (< 200 × 10$^9$/l), % | 12 | 20 |
| Leukaemic blood picture, % | 3 | 12 |
| ESR, mm/h | 71 (47) | 91 (50) |
| M-component (serum), g/l | 42/20 | 45/32 |
| IgG, % | 57 | 49 |
| IgA, % | 29 | 21 |
| IgG + A, % | 1 | 4 |
| IgD, % | – | 4 |
| IgE, % | – | 2 |
| Non-secretory, % | 13 | 18 |
| Bence Jones protein, % | 40 | 45 |
| Azotaemia (creatinine > 1.5 mg/dl), % | 15 | 34 |
| Hypercalcaemia (Ca > 5.5 val/l), % | 18 | 26 |
| Infiltration, vol% | 25 (19) | 44 (22) |
| Haematopoietic tissue, vol% | 22 (13) | 12 (11) |
| Fatty tissue, vol% | 27 (14) | 18 (15) |
| Sinusoids, vol% | 2 (1) | 2 (1) |
| Trabecular bone, vol% | 19 (6) | 20 (5) |
| Growth pattern |  |  |
|   Interstitial, % | 46 | 9 |
|   Myelomatous, % | 41 | 43 |
|   Packed marrow, % | 13 | 38 |
| Osteoblastic index[1] | 10 (12) | 11 (12) |
| Osteoclastic index[2] | 35 (25) | 46 (36) |
| Lymphoid nodules, % | 18 | 11 |

Numbers in parentheses = standard deviations.
[1] Percentage of trabecular circumference covered by cuboidal osteoblasts.
[2] Number of osteoclasts per 100 mm trabecular circumference.

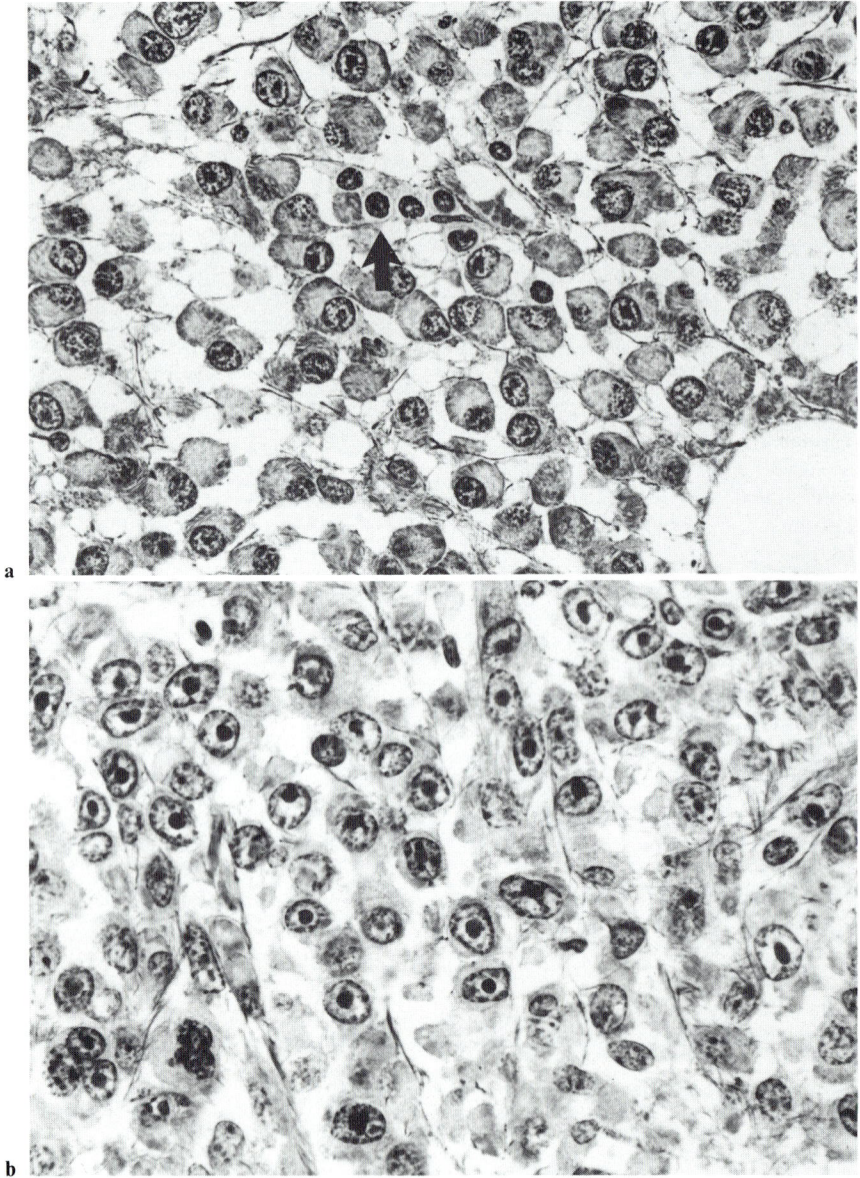

**Fig. 50.** Histologic types of MM in the bone marrow. Gomori. × 400. **a** MM plasmacytic, with mature plasma cells, some lymphocytes (→) and fine fibrosis. **b** MM plasmablastic, with predominantly nucleolated plasma cells and fine fibrosis.

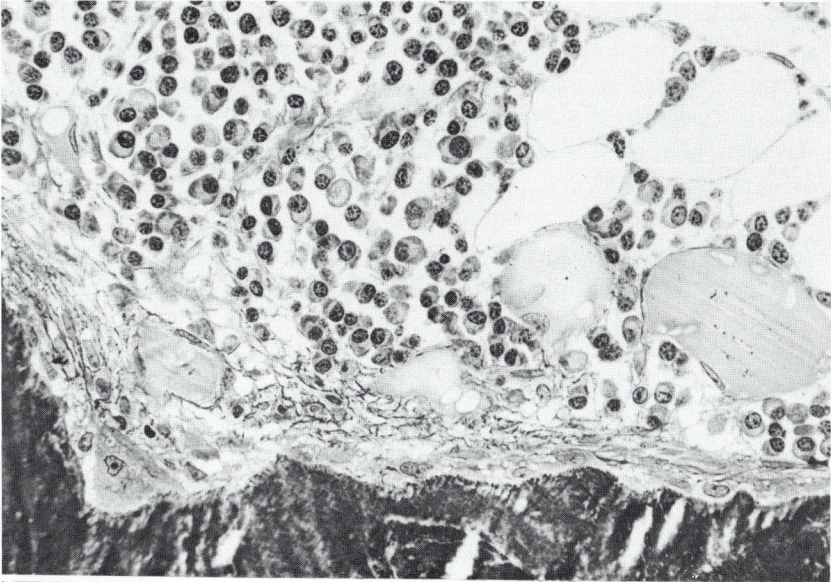

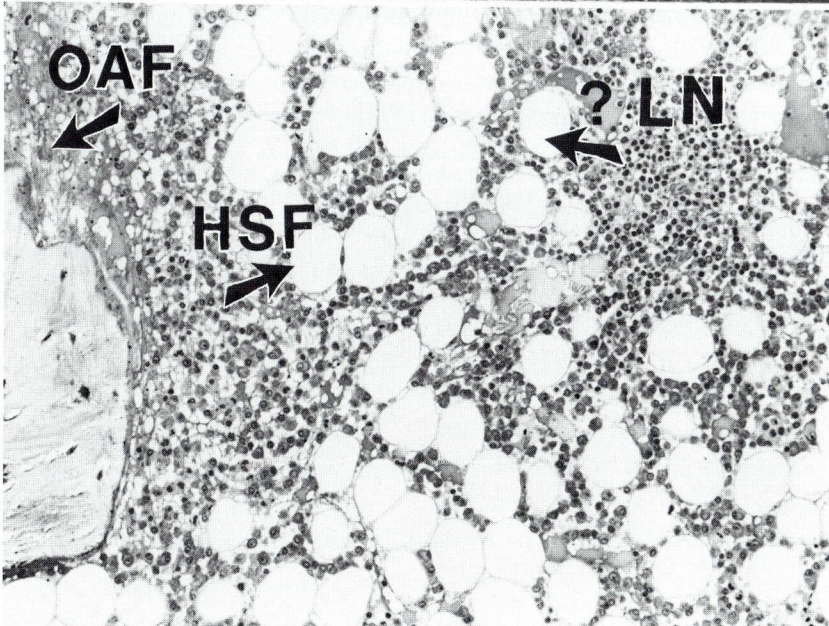

**Fig. 51.** Osteoclastic bone resorption in MM, plasmacytic type. Gomori. $\times 100$.

**Fig. 52.** Pathogenesis of increased osteoclastic bone resorption and of haematopoietic hypoplasia in MM. OAF = Osteoclast activating factor; HSF = haematopoiesis suppressing factor. Activated suppressor T lymphocytes may also suppress the haematopoietic tissue. LN = Lymphoid nodule. Giemsa. $\times 100$.

stitial, with dense perivascular and paratrabecular seams of myeloma cells, in 42% of the cases plasma cell aggregates, 'myelomas', were found in addition to the interstitial infiltration, and a complete replacement of the marrow, a packed marrow pattern, occurred in 18%. Small lymphocytic aggregates were seen in 15% of all cases, and all had a moderate increase in reticulin fibres. Additional histologic characteristics were fatty marrow atrophy and inhibition of erythropoiesis. Increased osteoclastic resorption and a pronounced rarefaction of the trabeculae were seen in most cases (fig. 51, 52). The median survival was 41 months from the onset of symptoms and 32 months from the time of the first biopsy. The prognostic significance of the myeloma cell burden in the biopsy (vol%) is shown in table X. Three stages were distinguished: stage I with less than 20 vol% (interstitial), stage II with 20–50 vol% (myelomatous) and stage III with more than 50 vol% (packed marrow). Statistical analysis of the survival times showed that these histologic stages corresponded to the progression of the disease (table X).

The *plasmablastic type* displayed a considerable polymorphism. Most cells were large, with clear round nuclei and distinct central nucleoli (fig. 50b). Multinucleated cells and a high mitotic rate were present in most cases. Some mature plasma cells, lymphocytes and immunoblasts were also scattered among the plasmablasts. The most frequent growth pattern was the packed marrow type, with marked reduction in fat cells and haemato-

**Table X.** Histologic classification and staging of MM in the bone marrow biopsy – median survival (months) at time of initial biopsy

| | |
|---|---|
| *Classification* | |
| Plasmacytic (n = 149) | 32 |
| Plasmablastic (n = 71) | 8 |
| *Staging* | |
| Plasmacytic | |
|     < 20 vol% | 36 |
|     20–50 vol% | 29 |
|     > 50 vol% | 16 |
| Plasmablastic | |
|     < 20 vol% | 21 |
|     20–50 vol% | 10 |
|     > 50 vol% | 5 |

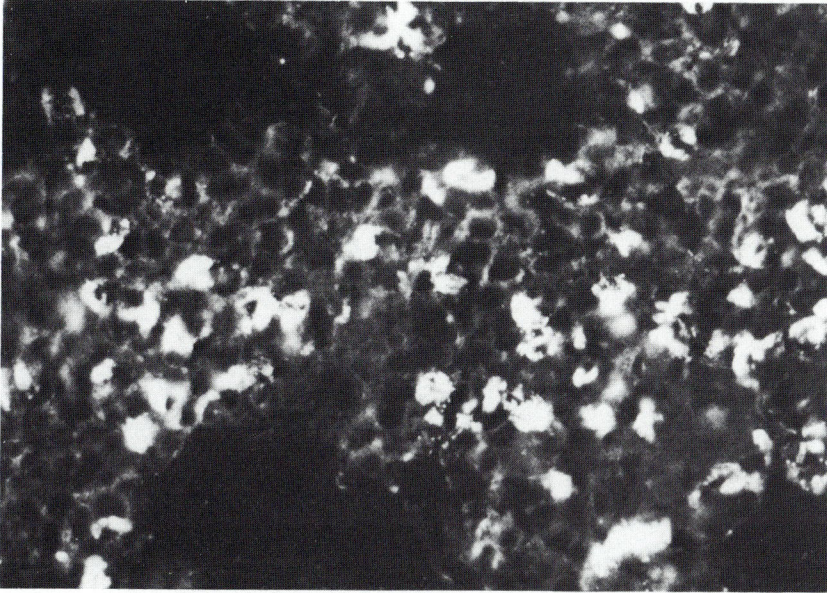

**Fig. 53.** Detection of an early stage of MM by immunohistology. Bone marrow cryo-stat section, FITC, anti-IgA. × 250.

poiesis. The median survival time from the onset of symptoms was 19 months, and 8 months from the time of the first biopsy. The patients in the plasmablastic group were also divided into three categories according to the volume percentages of infiltration in the biopsy. As in the plasmablastic type the three stages corresponded to the progression of the disease (table X).

## Implications for Medical Practice

In search for dependable diagnostic criteria some authors have already pointed out the contribution bone marrow biopsy can make to the diagnosis of MM [5, 6, 11, 36]. The findings presented above confirm their observations and demonstrate the diagnostic value of histologic and histomorphometric bone marrow data such as the growth patterns and the volume percentages of myeloma cells (tumour burden). Furthermore, immunohistologic evaluations of the bone marrow have been successfully applied to diagnose borderline cases (fig. 53) [6, 28].

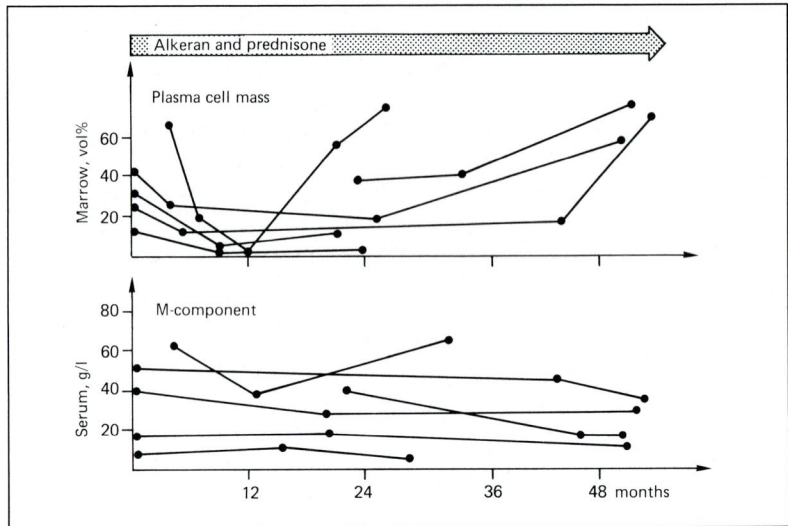

**Fig. 54.** Follow-up of the plasma cell mass in the biopsy and of the M-component (serum) under cytostatic therapy, investigated on 6 patients with MM.

Indirect indicators such as anaemia, hypercalcaemia or uraemia have previously been shown to have greater prognostic value than the more direct tumour-derived criteria such as type and level of the M component [1, 20, 21]. Our results have demonstrated that histologic parameters in the bone marrow (e.g. maturity of plasma cells, volume of plasma cell infiltration in the biopsy as well as proliferation pattern, mitotic activity and fibre content) have significant prognostic value. Moreover, it was shown that MM may be divided into a plasmacytic type of low-grade malignancy and a plasmablastic type of high-grade malignancy, analogous to NHL. Both types may be staged according to the volume percentages of the plasma cell infiltration in the biopsy: stage I < 20 vol%, stage II 20–50 vol% and stage III > 50 vol%. These stages correlated significantly with the patients' clinical histories and their survival times. *Durie and Salmon* [13] and *Durie* et al. [14] have proposed a three-stage system on the basis of the calculated myeloma cell burden. More recently, *Merlini* et al. [24] proposed a further three-stage system for MM based on statistical correlations between the clinical features and survival in 123 deceased patients. *Pennec* et al. [26] have tested the clinical value of different staging systems of MM. The information derived from the histologic evaluation of bone marrow biopsies can be utilized to supplement the clinical criteria for staging (fig. 54).

## References

1   Alexanian, R.; Balcerzak, S.; Bonnet, J.D.; Gehan, E.A.; Haut, A.; Hewlett, J.S.; Monto, R.W.: Prognostic factors in multiple myeloma. Cancer *36:* 1192–1201 (1975).

2   Apitz, K.: Die neuen Anschauungen vom Plasmozytom des Knochenmarks, dem sog. multiplen Myelom. Klin. Wschr. *40:* 1025–1029 (1940).

3   Astaldi, G.; Wuhrmann, F.; Wunderly, C.: Untersuchungen über Korrelation zwischen Proliferationstätigkeit, cytologischem Bild, Para-Dysproteinämie und klinischem Verlauf des Plasmocytoms. Klin. Wschr. *32:* 139–140 (1954).

4   Azar, H.A.; Potter, M.: Multiple myeloma and related disorders, vol. I (Harper & Row, Hagerstown 1973).

5   Bartl, R.; Burkhardt, R.; Gierster, P.; Sandel, P.; Fateh-Moghadam, A.: Significance of bone marrow biopsy in the multiple myeloma; in Ulutin, Recent progress in cell biology: leukocytes and platelets. Biblthca haemat., vol. 45, pp. 81–86 (Karger, Basel 1978).

6   Bartl, R.; Frisch, B.; Burkhardt, R.; Fateh-Moghadam, A.; Gierster, P.; Sund, M.; Kettner, G.: Bone marrow histology in myeloma: its importance in diagnosis, prognosis, classification and staging. Br. J. Haemat. *51:* 371–375 (1982).

7   Bataille, R.: Localized plasmacytomas. Clin. Haematol. *11:* 113–122 (1982).

8   Bayrd, E.D.: The bone marrow on sternal aspiration in multiple myeloma. Blood *3:* 987–1018 (1948).

9   Beer, F.; Martin, J.; Steffen, C.: Morphologische und klinisch-chemische Prognosestellung bei Plasmocytomen. Klin. Med. *9:* 207–215 (1954).

10  Buckman, R.; Cuzick, J.; Galton, D.A.G.: Long-term survival in myelomatosis. A report to the MRC Working Party on leucaemia in adults. Br. J. Haematol. *52:* 589–599 (1982).

11  Canale, D.D.; Collins, R.D.: Use of bone marrow particle sections in the diagnosis of multiple myeloma. Am. J. clin. Path. *61:* 383–392 (1974).

12  Corwin, J.; Lindberg, R.D.: Solitary plasmacytoma of bone vs. extramedullary plasmacytoma and their relationship to multiple myeloma. Cancer *43:* 1007–1013 (1979).

13  Durie, B.G.M.; Salmon, S.E.: Multiple myeloma, macroglobulinaemia, and monoclonal gammopathies; in Hoffbrand, Brain, Hirsh, Recent advances in haematology, vol. 2 (Churchill Livingstone, London 1977).

14  Durie, B.G.M.; Salmon, S.Y.; Moon, T.E.: Pretreatment tumor mass, cell kinetics, and prognosis in multiple myeloma. Blood *55:* 364–372 (1980).

15  Durie, B.G.M.; Salmon, S.E.; Mundy, G.R.: Relation of osteoclast activating factor production to extent of bone disease in multiple myeloma. Br. J. Haemat. *47:* 21–30 (1981).

16  Fateh-Moghadam, A.: Paraproteinämische Hämoblastosen; in Begemann, Handbuch der inneren Medizin; 5. Aufl., vol. II/5, pp. 24–252 (Springer, Berlin 1974).

17  Kapadia, S.B.: Multiple myeloma: a clinicopathologic study of 62 consecutively autopsied cases. Medicine, Baltimore *59:* 380–392 (1980).

18  Kiang, D.I.; Sundberg, R.D.; Fortuny, I.E.; Brunning, R.D.; Theologides, A.; Goldman, A.; Kennedy, B.J.: Multiple myeloma: clinical evolution. Minn. Med. *57:* 542–548 (1974).

19   Kyle, R.A.: Long-term survival in multiple myeloma. New Engl. J. Med. *308:* 314–316 (1983).

20   Kyle, R.A.; Bayrd, E.D.: The monoclonal gammopathies. Multiple myeloma and related plasma cell disorders (Thomas, Springfield 1976).

21   Kyle, R.A.; Elveback, L.R.: Management and prognosis of multiple myeloma. Mayo Clin. Proc. *51:* 751–760 (1976).

22   Kyle, R.A.; Greipp, P.R.: Smoldering multiple myeloma. New Engl. J. Med. *302:* 1347–1349 (1980).

23   Mellstedt, H.; Pettersson, D.; Holm, G.: Monoclonal B-lymphocytes in peripheral blood of patients with plasma cell myeloma. Scand. J. Haematol. *16:* 112–120 (1976).

24   Merlini, G.; Waldenström, J.G.; Jayakar, S.D.: A new improved clinical staging system for multiple myeloma based on analysis of 123 treated patients. Blood *55:* 1011–1019 (1980).

25   Paredes, J.M.; Mitchell, B.S.: Multiple myeloma. Current concepts in diagnosis and management. Med. Clins N. Am. *64:* 729–742 (1980).

26   Pennec, Y.; Mottier, D.; Youinou, P.; Asselain, B.; Chavance, M.; Legoff, P.; Leprise, P.-Y.; Miossec, P.; Lemenn, G.: Critical study of staging in multiple myeloma. Scand. J. Haematol. *30:* 183–190 (1983).

27   Petterson, D.; Mellstedt, H.; Holm, G.; Björkholm, M.: Monoclonal blood lymphocytes in benign monoclonal gammopathy and multiple myeloma, in relation to clinical stage. Scand. J. Haematol. *27:* 287–293 (1981).

28   Pizzolo, G.; Chilosi, M.; Cetto, G.L.; Fiore-Donati, L.; Janossy, G.: Immuno-histological analysis of bone marrow involvement in lymphoproliferative disorders. Br. J. Haemat. *50:* 95–100 (1982).

29   Rowan, R.M.: Multiple myeloma: some recent developments. Clin. Lab. Haemat. *4:* 211–230 (1982).

30   Salmon, S.E.: Immunoglobulin synthesis and tumor kinetics of multiple myeloma. Semin. Hematol. *10:* 135–147 (1973).

31   Snapper, I.; Kahn, A.: Myelomatosis. Fundamentals and clinical features (Karger, Basel 1971).

32   Stavem, P.; Førre, Ø.: The same type of crystalline inclusions in T-lymphocytes as in plasma cells and B-lymphocytes in multiple myeloma. Scand. J. Haematol. *26:* 265–271 (1981).

33   Valentin-Opran, A.; Charhon, S.A.; Meunier, P.J.; Edouard, C.M.; Arlot, M.E.: Quantitative histology of myeloma-induced bone changes. Br. J. Haemat. *52:* 601–610 (1982).

34   Vercelli, D.; Di Guglielmo, R.; Guidi, G.; Scolari, L.; Buricchi, L.; Cozzolino, F.: Bone marrow percentage of plasma cells in the staging of monoclonal gammopathies. Nouv. Revue fr. Hémat. *22:* 139–145 (1980).

35   Vercelli, D.; Cozzolino, F.; Di Guglielmo, R.: A comparison of two staging systems for myeloma. Nouv. Revue fr. Hémat. *23:* 107–110 (1981).

36   Wutke, K.; Varbiro, M.; Rüdiger, K.D.; Kelenyi, G.: Cytological and histological classification of multiple myeloma. Haematologia *14:* 315–329 (1981).

# 7  Non-Hodgkin's Lymphomas (NHL)

## Survey of the Literature

During the past decade the malignant lymphomas have been the subject of intense interest and activity resulting in great progress in the management of Hodgkin's disease. The situation with respect to the heterogenous group of NHL is less favourable [31]. The term NHL has established itself through widespread usage and encompasses a whole range of clinical and morphologic entities. At present there is no general agreement of the histologic classification of these morphologically diverse tumours [1, 2, 18, 26, 29, 35].

The first classification, introduced by *Rappaport* [28] in 1966, has been widely adopted in practice, in spite of its considerable heterogeneity. *Lukes and Collins* [24] have proposed a classification based on the identification of B and T lymphocytes and lymphocytic transformation. A functional interpretation of the NHL was developed independently by *Lennert* and coworkers [21, 22]. Both classifications stress the fact that the majority of NHL are tumours of B cell origin [20].

Bone marrow biopsy is considered as an integral part of initial diagnosis in NHL [11, 13, 15]. *Rosenberg* [30] showed that almost half of the NHL patients had bone marrow manifestations on first presentation, and this has been confirmed by other centres. A survey of the literature over the past decade shows a wide range (16–73%) in the incidence of bone marrow involvement [4, 5, 12, 16]. Various factors may be implicated to account for this considerable disparity: (1) the use of aspiration, which has a high rate of false negatives, (2) the non-uniformity of definitions for the NHL leading to varying distribution of patients in each category, (3) the unequal proportions of patients with early and advanced disease in the studies reported, and (4) the fact that biopsy size, site and technical preparation differ between reporting centres [13, 15].

The three classifications mentioned above are based on lymph node histology. But as lymph nodes are not always readily available, in some cases the histologic diagnosis must be made on material from other sites [5]. There are few studies on whether the criteria of lymph node histology are applicable and prognostically significant in other sites also. Though the histologic findings of NHL in the bone marrow have been described, and *Georgii* [17] has applied the Kiel classification to bone marrow histology, the reproducibility and the prognostic significance of such a classification were not investigated in those studies. This lack is somewhat surprising in view of the high incidence of bone marrow involvement in NHL. In this study on bone marrow histology, Lennert's nomenclature, which is widely employed in Europe, was used to enable comparison of lymph node and bone marrow findings in NHL.

## Own Observations

A total of 670 patients with NHL was investigated; none had received specific therapy prior to the first bone marrow biopsy. Patients with chronic lymphocytic leukaemia (CLL) were included, those with acute lymphocytic leukaemia (ALL) were excluded from this series. Sequential biopsies for restaging were obtained in 104 patients, and survival data were available for all 670 patients.

### Definition and Incidence of Bone Marrow Involvement

Benign lymphoid nodules [19, 33] are relatively frequent in bone marrow biopsies (found in 8% of our 25,000 biopsies) [3, 5, 9] and must be differentiated from lymphomatous infiltration (fig. 55, 56). Identification of lymphoid nodules as benign was usually not difficult, but problems did arise when they were large (more than 1 mm in diameter) and/or numerous. In 6 cases a second biopsy was required a few months later to establish the correct diagnosis. The distinction between monoclonal and reactive lymphocytic aggregates is possible by means of immunohistology on cryostat sections of bone marrow biopsies.

Bone marrow involvement was found in 465 of the 670 pretreatment patients with NHL, an overall incidence of 69% (table XI). The initial histologic diagnosis of NHL was established by bone marrow histology in 170 patients, corresponding to 25% of the NHL patients investigated. Patients with NHL of low-grade malignancy had a significantly higher incidence of bone marrow involvement than those with NHL of high-grade malignancy (77 and 26%, respectively), as shown in table XI.

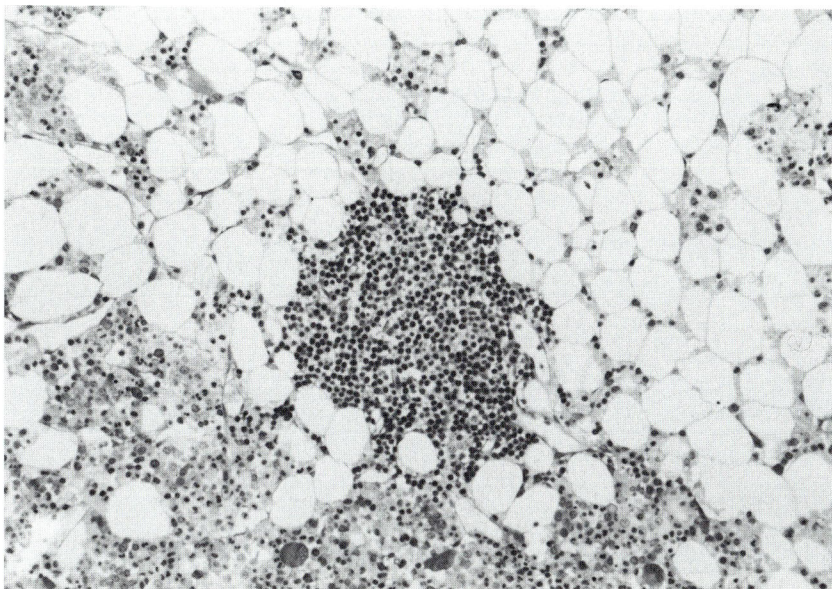

**Fig. 55.** Benign lymphoid nodule in the bone marrow. Gallamin blue-Giemsa. × 100.

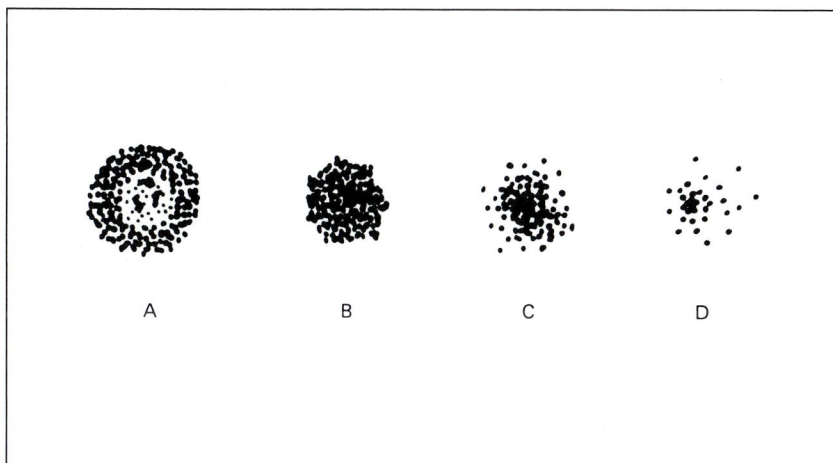

**Fig. 56.** Benign lymphoid nodules in the bone marrow. A = Nodules with germinal centres (5 %); B = sharply demarkated nodules (40 %); C = well defined nodules (40 %); D = small aggregates of lymphocytes (15 %).

**Table XI.** Frequency of bone marrow involvement in NHL (pretreatment patients)

| Histologic type | Positive biopsies, % |
|---|---|
| Lymphocytic | 99 |
| Hairy cell | 95 |
| Lymphoplasmacytic/cytoid | 85 |
| Centrocytic | 71 |
| Centroblastic/centrocytic | 20 |
| NHL of low-grade malignancy | 77 |
| Lymphoblastic (without ALL) | 39 |
| Immunoblastic | 22 |
| Centroblastic | 27 |
| Unclassifiable | 24 |
| NHL of high-grade malignancy | 26 |
| NHL overall | 69 |

## Identification of Prognostic Factors in Bone Marrow Histology

9 histologic parameters were assessed for their predictive value. The simplest and most reliable criterion for categorizing NHL in the bone marrow proved to be the growth pattern. Four distinct patterns were recognized: interstitial, 'packed marrow', nodular, and paratrabecular (fig. 57). Statistic analysis showed that the patients with nodular marrow involvement had significantly longer survivals than those with the other three patterns. Patients with a 'packed marrow' pattern constituted the most unfavourable group (table XII, fig. 58). The presence of germinal centres was also a significant favourable factor, though their occurrence was linked to the nodular pattern. A large tumour cell burden (vol%) in the bone marrow biopsy correlated significantly with short survival times. However, the maturity of the proliferative cell system constituted the most significant prognostic factor of NHL in the bone marrow. Patients in the 'mature cell group', characterized by predominantly non-nucleolated cells, had far longer survivals than those in the 'immature cell group', with predominantly nucleolated cells. Each type of NHL (Kiel classification) was separately correlated with duration of survival: the prognostic relevance is documented in

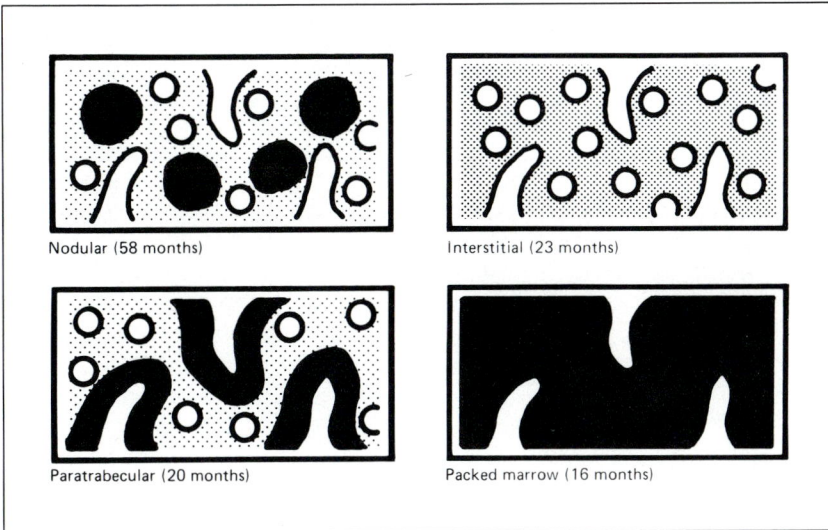

Fig. 57. Patterns of NHL in the bone marrow histology and their prognostic relevance (median survival time).

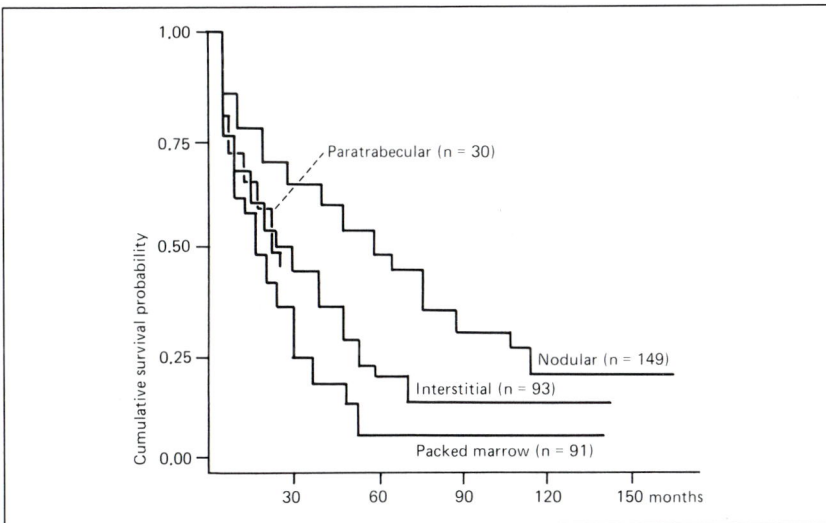

Fig. 58. Predictive value of bone marrow histology in NHL; grouping variable is 'growth pattern'.

**Table XII.** Prognostic factors of NHL in the bone marrow biopsy

| Histologic criteria | Patients | Median survival months | Breslow, Mantel-Cox p values |
|---|---|---|---|
| Proliferative cell system | | | 0.0001 |
|   Lymphocytic | 132 | 41 | 0.0001 |
|   Hairy cell | 87 | 21 | |
|   Immunocytic | 90 | 44 | |
|   Centrocytic | 20 | 25 | |
|   Centroblastic/cytic | 17 | 50 | |
|   Immunoblastic | 13 | 4 | |
|   Centroblastic | 7 | 5 | |
|   Unclassifiable | 4 | 5 | |
| Cell maturity | | | 0.0001 |
|   Mature | 364 | 36 | 0.0001 |
|   Immature | 24 | 5 | |
| Growth pattern | | | 0.0001 |
|   Nodular | 149 | 58 | 0.0001 |
|   Interstitial | 93 | 23 | |
|   Paratrabecular | 30 | 20 | |
|   Packed marrow | 91 | 16 | |
| Infiltration | | | 0.0005 |
|   $< 20$ vol% | 110 | 73 | 0.0001 |
|   20–50 vol% | 121 | 30 | |
|   $> 50$ vol% | 133 | 24 | |
| Mitotic activity | | | 0.0002 |
|   Low | 332 | 37 | 0.0001 |
|   High | 38 | 6 | |
| Cellular atypia | | | 0.0039 |
|   Low | 312 | 38 | 0.0013 |
|   High | 58 | 18 | |
| Fibrosis | | | 0.0002 |
|   Fine | 319 | 36 | 0.0003 |
|   Coarse | 50 | 11 | |
| Stromal reaction | | | 0.0134 |
|   Low | 229 | 37 | 0.0051 |
|   High | 141 | 29 | |
| Bone remodelling | | | 0.0041 |
|   Normal | 350 | 29 | 0.0031 |
|   Increased | 19 | 9 | |

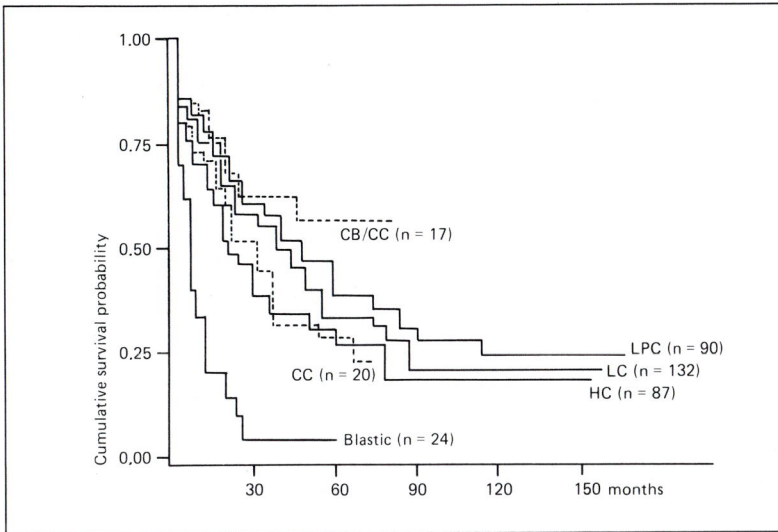

**Fig. 59.** Predictive value of bone marrow histology in NHL; grouping variable is 'proliferative cell system'. CB/CC = Centroblastic/centrocytic; CC = centrocytic; HC = hairy cell; LC = lymphocytic; LPC = lymphoplasmacytic/cytoid.

the survival curves in figure 59. A high mitotic rate and a pronounced cellular polymorphism indicated significantly shorter survivals. Non-specific bone marrow changes such as fibrosis, osseous remodelling and stromal reactions within the neoplastic infiltrations also appeared to have some prognostic value (table XII).

*Histologic Classification*
Bone marrow biopsies were classified as follows (fig. 60; table XIII):

Malignant Lymphomas (ML) of Low-Grade Malignancy
*ML Lymphocytic.* The bone marrow was characterized by infiltration with typical small lymphocytes and a few prolymphocytes and lympho-

---

**Fig. 60** (on p. 78 and 79). Histologic types of NHL in the bone marrow. Gallamin blue-Giemsa. × 250. **a** ML lymphocytic. **b** ML hairy cell. **c** ML lymphoplasmacytic/cytoid. **d** ML centrocytic. **e** ML centroblastic/centrocytic. **f** ML centroblastic. **g** ML lymphoblastic. **h** ML immunoblastic.

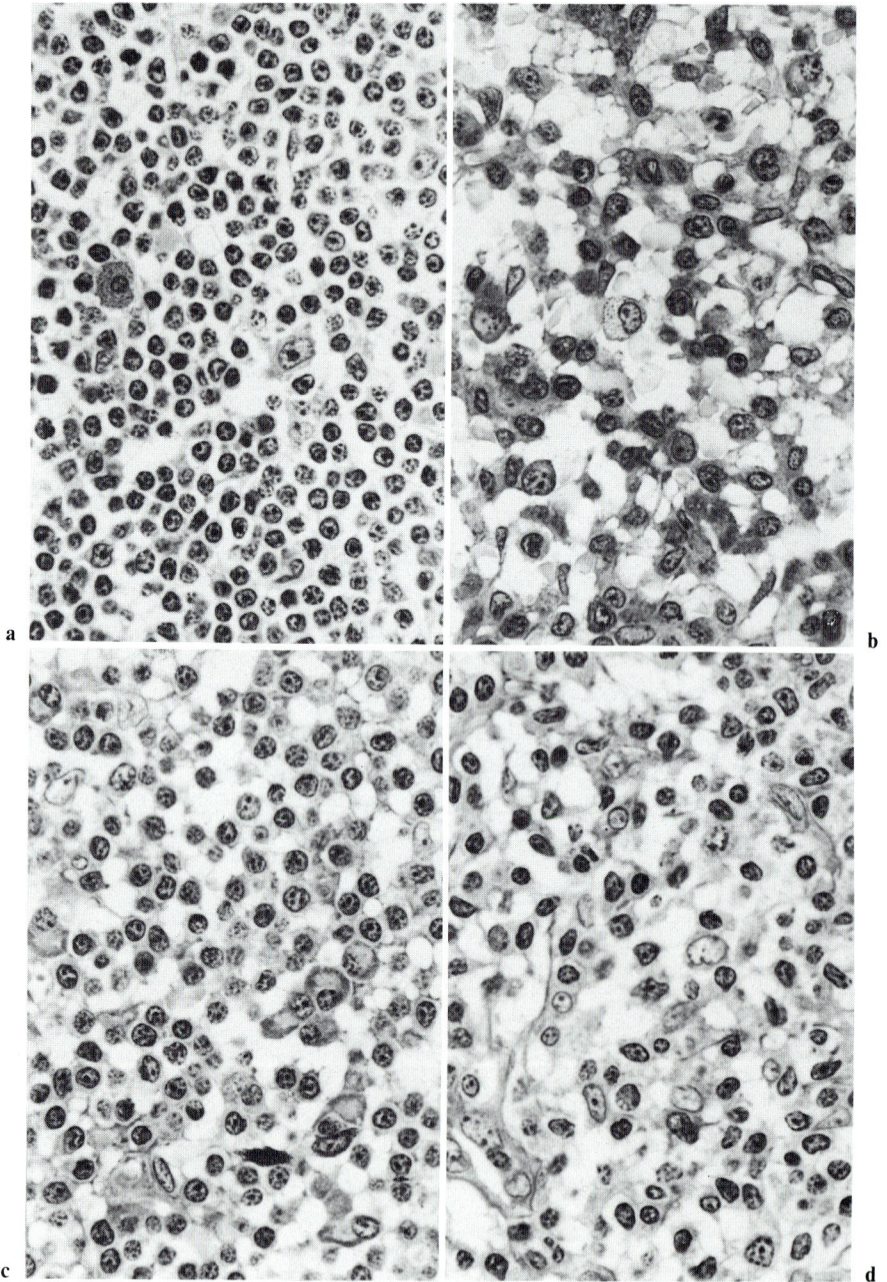

**Fig. 60.** Legend p. 77.

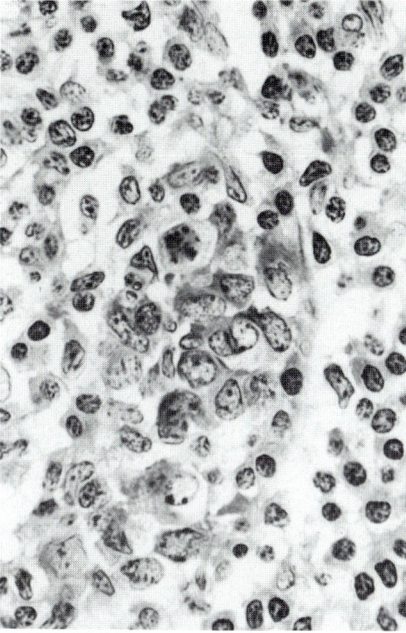

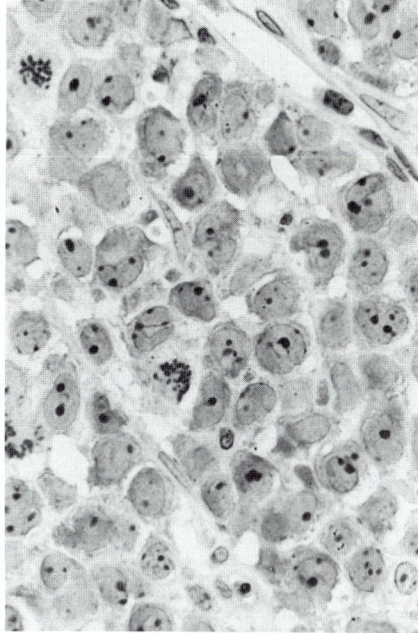

e

f

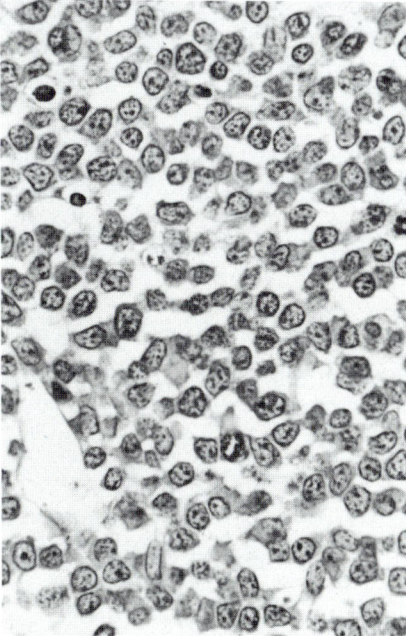

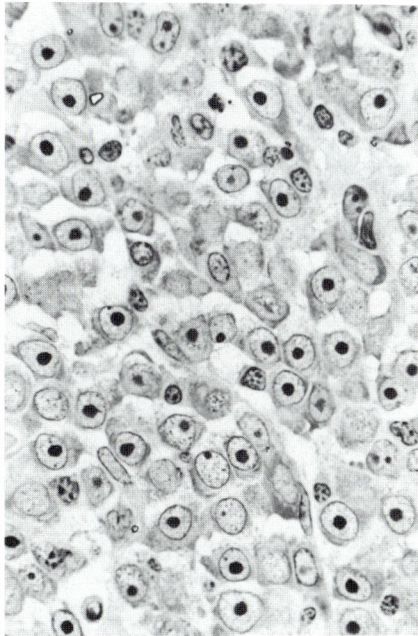

g

h

**Table XIII.** Histologic classification of NHL in the bone marrow – 366 untreated patients at time of initial biopsy

| | Lymphocytic | Hairy cell | Immunocytic | Centrocytic | Centroblastic/ centrocytic | Blastic (without ALL) |
|---|---|---|---|---|---|---|
| Patients | 132 | 87 | 90 | 20 | 17 | 20 |
| Male/female | 1.2 | 3.2 | 1.2 | 1.3 | 1.1 | 1.4 |
| Age, median, years | 65 | 52 | 63 | 58 | 60 | 49 |
| Lymphomas | 69 | 8 | 34 | 58 | 42 | 40 |
| Splenomegaly ≤ 5 cm b.c.m., % | 30 | 39 | 19 | 30 | 19 | 23 |
| Splenomegaly > 5 cm b.c.m., % | 26 | 40 | 38 | 22 | 19 | 19 |
| Hepatomegaly, % | 47 | 47 | 34 | 39 | 30 | 38 |
| Anaemia (Hb <10 g/dl), % | 18 | 65 | 28 | 32 | 8 | 46 |
| Leukopenia (<4 × 10⁹/l), % | 2 | 22 | 20 | 14 | 16 | 18 |
| Leukocytosis (>10 × 10⁹/l), % | 88 | 8 | 14 | 25 | 5 | 20 |
| Leukaemic blood picture, % | 98 | 70 | 8 | 25 | 5 | 21 |
| Thrombopenia (<100 × 10⁹/l), % | 36 | 85 | 28 | 30 | 22 | 34 |
| Infiltration, vol% | 43 (20) | 48 (15) | 30 (20) | 43 (21) | 15 (20) | 58 (12) |
| Infiltration <20 vol%, % | 14 | 7 | 39 | 21 | 76 | 14 |
| Haematopoietic tissue, vol% | 15 (12) | 12 (11) | 25 (20) | 15 (10) | 30 (18) | 8 (4) |
| Fatty tissue, vol% | 13 (14) | 8 (5) | 9 (10) | 13 (13) | 31 (18) | 7 (10) |
| Sinusoids, vol% | 2 (1) | 6 (4) | 4 (3) | 2 (2) | 3 (1) | 2 (2) |
| Trabecular bone, vol% | 22 (6) | 20 (4) | 24 (6) | 24 (6) | 22 (4) | 25 (6) |
| Growth pattern | | | | | | |
| Interstitial, % | 42 | 0 | 4 | 0 | 0 | 0 |
| Interstitial/nodular, % | 32 | 0 | 34 | 0 | 0 | 0 |
| Nodular, % | 0 | 0 | 38 | 0 | 80 | 0 |
| Paratrabecular, % | 0 | 0 | 0 | 60 | 0 | 0 |
| Patchy, % | 0 | 75 | 0 | 0 | 0 | 0 |
| Packed marrow, % | 26 | 25 | 24 | 40 | 20 | 100 |
| Germinal centres, % | 25 | 0 | 29 | 0 | 86 | 0 |

b.c.m. = Below costal margin; numbers in parentheses = standard deviations.

blasts [4]. There was little reticulin (fig. 64e). Three patterns were observed: interstitial, 'packed marrow' and nodular; in 35% of these biopsies germinal centres were found in the nodules. Nearly all (99%) of the patients had a leukaemic blood picture and the clinical features of CLL. The median survival of the whole group was 43 months, though patients with the nodular bone marrow pattern had significantly longer survivals than in the other two groups (median survivals of 115 and 34 months, respectively). Additional prognostic factors were the infiltration volume percentage, the amount of nucleolated cells and the degree of nuclear clefts [27] (fig. 61). The immunologic differentiation of CLL can be performed by immunohistochemistry on frozen sections of the bone marrow biopsy (fig. 62).

*ML Hairy Cell.* The salient histologic bone marrow characteristic was a patchy to extensive replacement of the haematopoietic tissue by the typical hairy cells: lymphoid elements slightly larger than lymphocytes, with broader, often elongated rims of cytoplasm, bean-shaped, oval, round or cleaved nuclei with moderate amounts of heterochromatin. Three cytologic types of hairy cells were discernible, each of them with different prognostic relevance: 'ovoid', 'convoluted' and 'indented' [6]. 45% of the cases had histologically evident cytoplasmic inclusions (fig. 64a). The infiltration also contains plasma cells, lymphocytes and mast cells, all within a slightly inforced reticulin network. Extravasation of erythrocytes was consistently observed. Previous attempts at bone marrow aspiration had generally resulted in a 'dry tap', and the diagnosis was established in 90% of the cases by the bone marrow biopsy. The median survival time was 21 months and the extent of the infiltration in the bone marrow had prognostic significance.

*ML Lymphoplasmacytic/Cytoid (LP, Immunocytoma).* The bone marrow infiltration consisted primarily of small lymphocytes plus plasmacytoid cells, plasma cells and some mast cells [7]. Few nucleolated lymphoid cells were observed, there was little reticulin and about 33% of the cases had PAS-positive cytoplasmic or nuclear inclusions (fig. 64b, c). A nodular configuration occurred in 38%, a nodular plus interstitial pattern in 34% and a diffuse (interstitial and packed marrow type without nodules) in 28%. On the basis of the proportion of infiltrating cells, three subgroups were identified: (a) lymphoplasmacytoid (50% of the cases), with primarily small plasmacytoid cells and a nodular distribution; (b) lymphoplasmacytic (46% of the cases), with small lymphocytes plus typical plasma cells and mast cells, with a diffuse distribution; and (c) polymorphous (4% of the cases), consist-

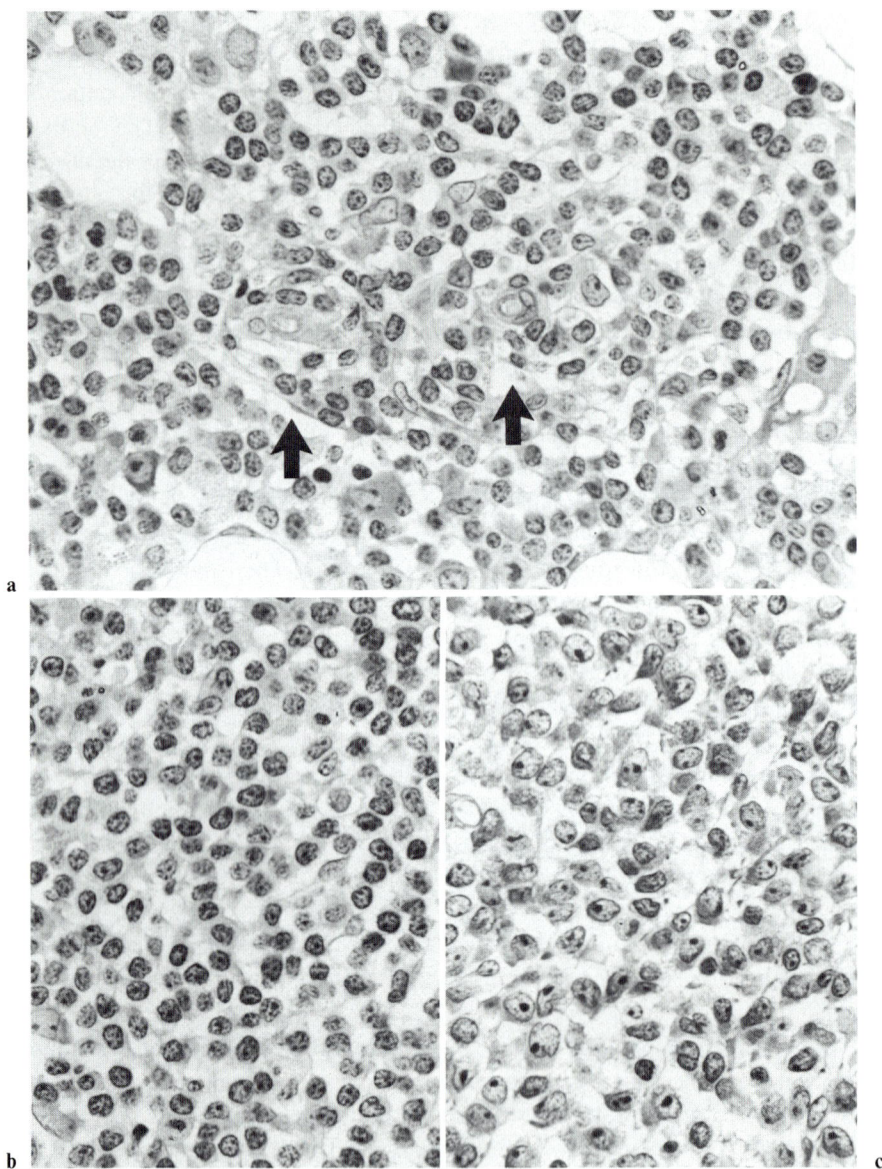

**Fig. 61. a** T-CLL with marked perivascular infiltration (arrows). Giemsa. × 400. **b** B2-CLL with cleaved nuclei of lymphocytes. Giemsa. × 400. **c** T-IB with nuclear polymorphism of the immunoblasts. Giemsa. × 400.

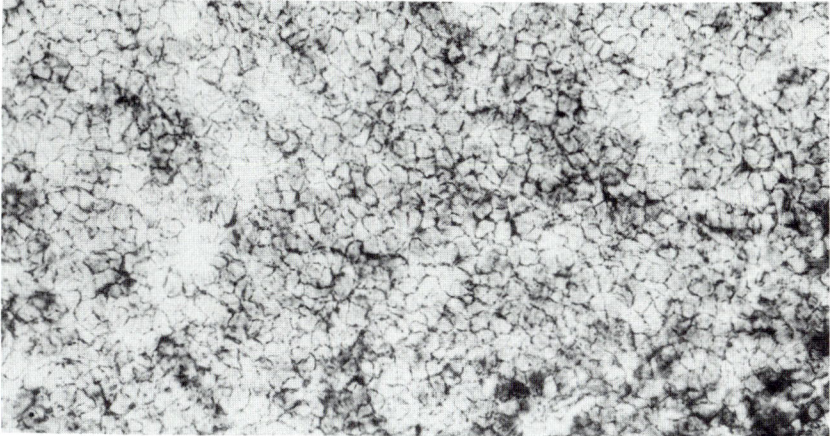

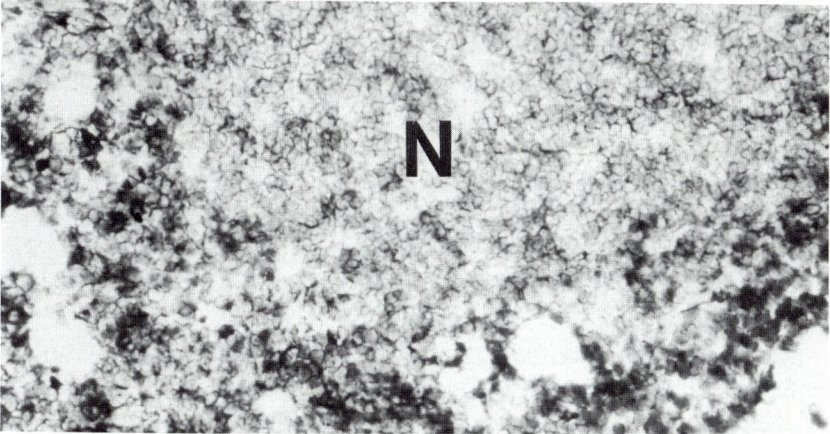

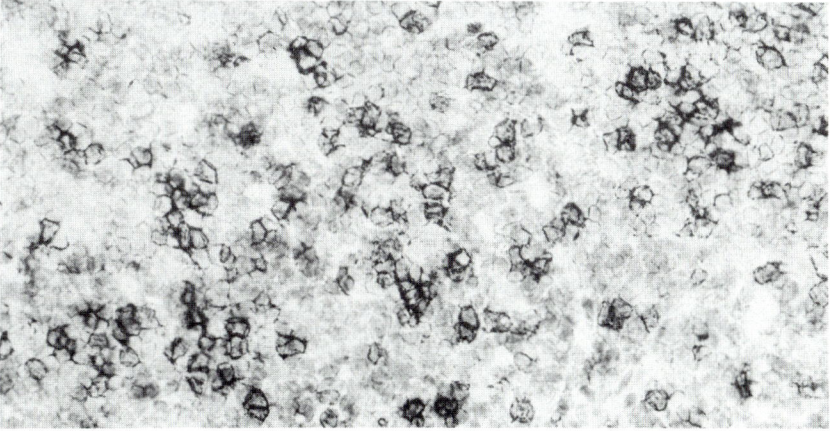

**Fig. 62.** Legend p. 84.

ing of a heterogenous lymphoid population (lymphocytes, centrocytes, centroblasts, immunoblasts) and plasma cells with a diffuse to a packed marrow growth pattern.

89% of all cases had an IgM-paraproteinaemia. Though there was a median survival of 44 months for the whole group, there were differences between the subgroups: lymphoplasmacytoid 63 months, lymphoplasmacytic 31 months and polymorphous 12 months. A greater or lesser extent of infiltration also had prognostic value (fig. 63).

*ML Centrocytic.* The infiltrating lymphoid cells in this lymphoma were characterized as small or large when their nuclei were smaller or larger than those of reactive histiocytes, and 'cleaved' when the nuclei were elongated or irregular with indentations or clefts. These cells had only narrow rims of cytoplasm. Variable numbers of non-cleaved lymphoid cells with one to three nucleoli (centroblasts) were also present. The infiltration was paratrabecular in 60% of the cases, 40% had a packed marrow pattern. There were predominantly small cleaved cells in 46%, large cleaved cells in 43% and polymorphous cells in 11%. The median overall survival was 28 months, with variations according to the cell type as follows: small cleaved (10 cases) 59 months, large cleaved (6 cases) 26 months and polymorphous (4 cases) 6 months. The volume percentage of infiltration also had a significant correlation with duration of survival.

*ML Centroblastic/Centrocytic.* Bone marrow involvement was strictly nodular. Many nodules were follicles with germinal centres (fig. 64d). The nodules contained lymphocytes, histiocytes, capillaries, arterioles, reticulin fibres as well as centrocytes and centroblasts. Further subtyping of the bone marrow manifestations in this ML was not possible. With 50 months, it had the longest median survival of all the ML with bone marrow involvement.

---

**Fig. 62.** Immunohistochemistry of bone marrow cryostat sections in CLL. × 210. **a** CLL, diffuse pattern: the majority of infiltrating lymphocytes is labelled by anti-kappa. PAP method. **b** CLL, nodular pattern. N = Lymphoid nodule composed of IgM-positive lymphocytes, surrounded by haematopoietic tissue with endogenous peroxidase activity. PAP method. **c** T lymphocytes distributed diffusely between negative neoplastic B-lymphocytes. Anti-T-globulin, PAP method.

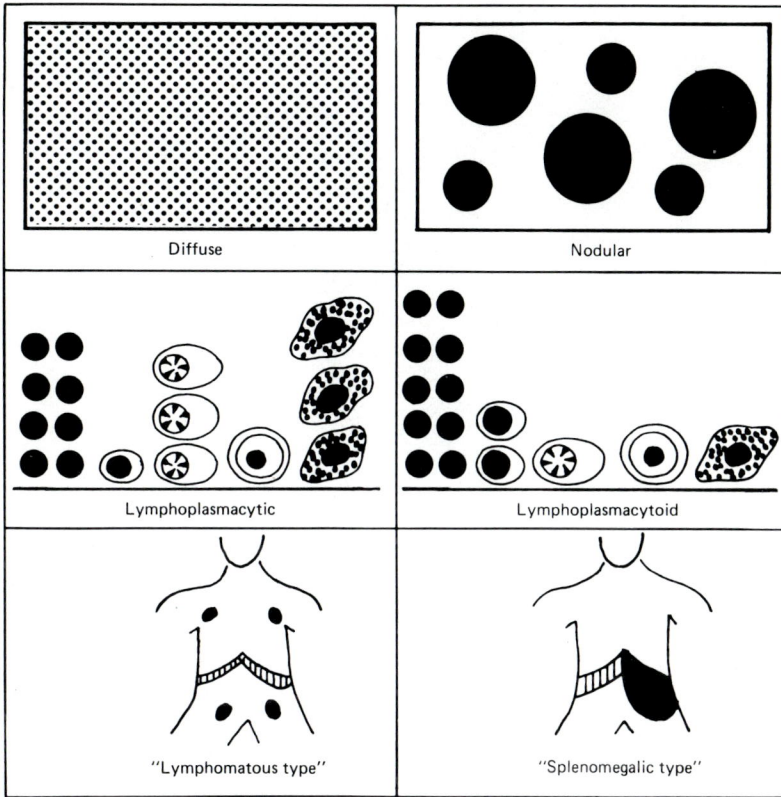

**Fig. 63.** Subtyping of immunocytoma according to the proliferation pattern and the proliferative cell system in the bone marrow.

Malignant Lymphomas of High-Grade Malignancy

The 28 patients in this group were classified as follows: immunoblastic 7, centroblastic 7, lymphoblastic (only sarcoma type) 10 and unclassifiable 4. But as the histologic features in the bone marrow were similar, they are grouped together. The identification of immunoblastic, centroblastic or lymphoblastic was made by cell size, nuclear chromatin and nucleoli. All 28 patients had a packed marrow type with an unfavourable prognosis, median survival of 5 months.

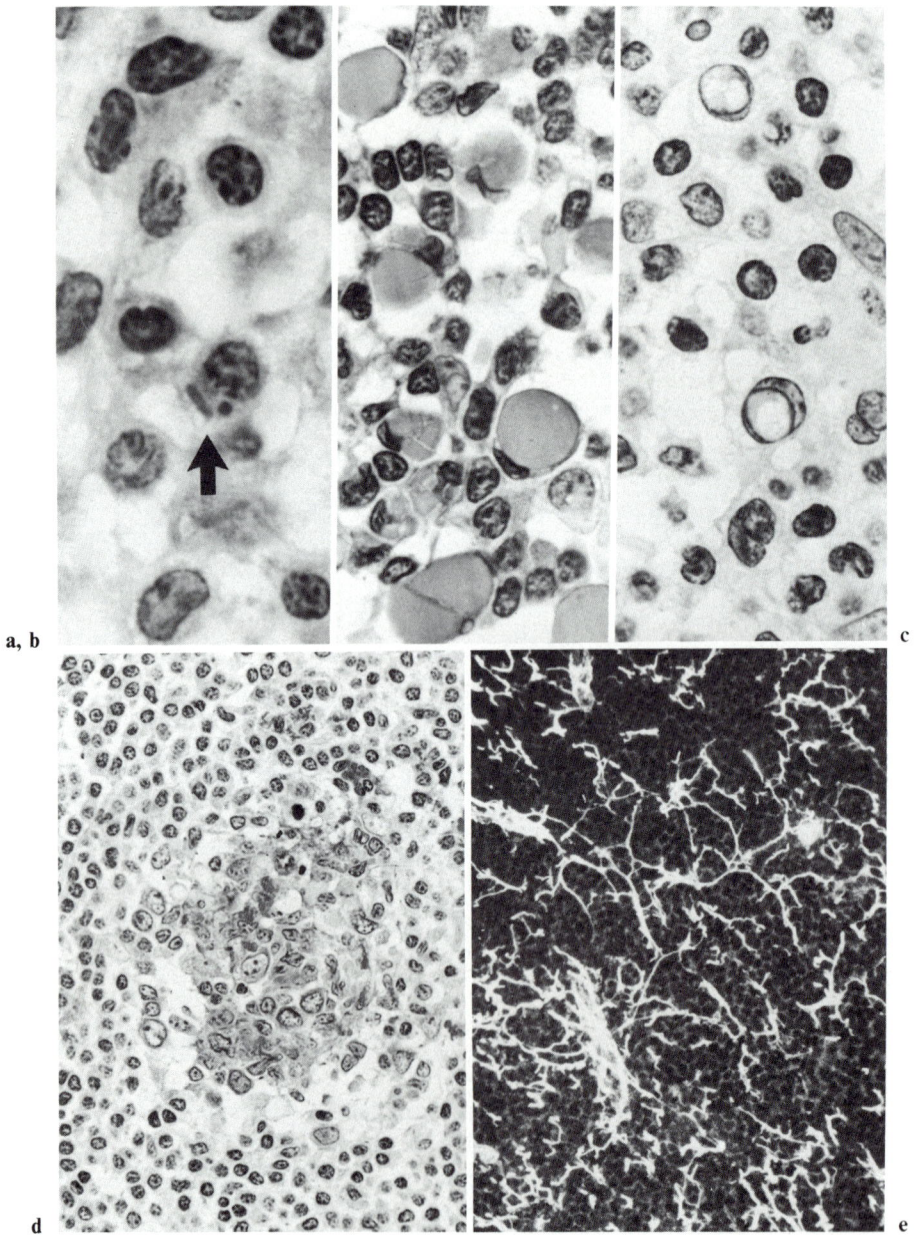

**Fig. 64. a** Rod-like inclusion bodies (arrow) in ML hairy cell. **b** Intracytoplasmic and **c** intranuclear inclusions in ML lymphoplasmacytic/cytoid. Gallamin blue-Giemsa. × 400.

## Implications for Medical Practice

In large series of patients investigated with adequate biopsy techniques, about half of all patients with NHL were found to have bone marrow infiltration at the time of initial diagnosis [5, 30]. Recently, *Chabner* et al. [11] demonstrated that the results of bone marrow biopsy placed 25% of unselected patients into stage IV. These observations have contributed to the decline of staging laparotomy in NHL. In our study the overall incidence was 69%, with a significantly higher incidence in the ML of low-grade than in those of high-grade malignancy (77 and 26%, respectively).

Our observations show that the Kiel classification can be applied to bone marrow manifestations, various aspects of which have prognostic relevance. The resulting survival curves were similar to those obtained on the basis of lymph node histology, but the patients classified by the bone marrow histology had somewhat shorter survivals [50]. The four growth patterns identified in the bone marrow also had predictive significance, and each type of NHL tended to one particular mode of spread. For example, CLL patients with a nodular pattern in the bone marrow had significantly longer survivals than those with a diffuse pattern [4, 9, 23, 32].

The Ann Arbor staging system proposed for both HD and NHL was widely adopted for HD but not for NHL, primarily due to differences in the mode of expansion and spread between the two disease groups [31]. Recent work with marker techniques has demonstrated that neoplastic lymphocytes circulate very early in the peripheral blood of patients with NHL and MM [1, 8, 34]. According to *Magrath* [25] bone marrow and peripheral blood involvement can occur especially in three groups of lymphoid neoplasms: (1) in neoplasms arising in stem cells normally resident in bone marrow, (2) in neoplasms in which the predominant cell normally migrates through blood and bone marrow, and (3) in neoplasms that arise in extraskeletal locations, with secondary involvement (metastases) of the bone marrow.

Viewed in this light, most NHL could well be considered as systemic diseases from the start so that the emphasis shifts from *whether* the bone

---

**d** Germinal centre in ML centroblastic/centrocytic. Gallamin blue-Giemsa. × 400. **e** Fine fibrosis, composed of collagen type III, in CLL. Frozen cryostat section, FITC, anti-collagen type III. × 250.

marrow is involved to the *extent* of its involvement, from *non-detectable* with routine methods [8] to *massive* infiltration. With respect to the bone marrow we distinguished three categories of expansion: (1) NHL with a primarily systemic presentation (e.g. CLL) – in these cases a useful criterion for staging proved to be the volume percentage of lymphoid infiltration in the bone marrow [4, 23, 32]; (2) NHL with a primarily regional presentation (e.g. centroblastic/centrocytic lymphoma) – in these cases there was mainly a centrifugal spread, comparable to HD, and a low incidence of bone marrow involvement, and (3) NHL with a metastatic behaviour (e.g. immunoblastic sarcoma) – there was an unpredictable pattern of spread analogous to a metastatic sarcoma.

These observations indicate conclusively that bone marrow biopsy is a useful diagnostic tool for histologic classification and clinical staging of any given patient with NHL.

## References

1   Aisenberg, A.C.: Cell lineage in lymphoproliferative disease. Am. J. Med. *74:* 679–685 (1983).
2   Bain, G.O.: Non-Hodgkin's lymphomas. Analysis of 92 cases using the 'international' classification. Archs Pathol. Lab. Med. *107:* 64–69 (1983).
3   Bartl, R.; Burkhardt, R.; Schlag, R.; Hill, W.: Nodular lymphoid hyperplasia and malignant lymphoma in the bone marrow biopsy in advanced age. 6th Meet. Int. Soc. Haematol., Eur. Afr. Div., Athens 1981.
4   Bartl, R.; Frisch, B.; Burkhardt, R.; Hoffmann-Fezer, G.; Demmler, K.; Sund, M.: Assessment of marrow trephine in relation to staging in chronic lymphocytic leukaemia. Br. J. Haemat. *51:* 1–15 (1982).
5   Bartl, R.; Frisch, B.; Burkhardt, R.; Kettner, G.; Fateh-Moghadam, A.; Sund, M.: Assessment of bone marrow histology in the malignant lymphomas (non-Hodgkin's). Correlation with clinical factors. Br. J. Haemat. *51:* 511–530 (1982).
6   Bartl, R.; Frisch, B.; Hill, W.; Burkhardt, R.; Sommerfeld, W.; Sund, M.: Bone marrow histology in hairy cell leukemia: identification of subtypes and their prognostic significance. Am. J. clin. Path. *79:* 531–545 (1983).
7   Bartl, R.; Frisch, B.; Mahl, G.; Burkhardt, R.; Fateh-Moghadam, A.; Pappenberger, R.; Sommerfeld, W.; Hoffmann-Fezer, G.: Bone marrow histology in Waldenström's macroglobulinaemia. Clinical relevance of subtype recognition. Scand. J. Haematol. *31:* 359–375 (1983).
8   Benjamin, D.; Magrath, I.T.; Douglass, E.C.; Corash, L.M.: Derivation of lymphoma cell lines from microscopically normal bone marrow in patients with undifferentiated lymphomas: evidence of occult bone marrow involvement. Blood *5:* 1017–1019 (1983).
9   Burkhardt, R.; Frisch, B.; Bartl, R.: Bone biopsy in haematological disorders. J. clin. Path. *35:* 257–284 (1982).

10    Brunning, R.D.; McKenna, R.W.: Bone marrow manifestations of malignant
      lymphoma and lymphoma-like conditions; in Sommers, Rosen, Pathology annual
      1979, part I, pp. 1–59 (Appleton-Century-Crofts, New York 1979).
11    Chabner, B.A.; Fisher, F.J.; Young, R.C.; Vita, V.T. de: Staging of non-Hodgkin's
      lymphomas; in Coltman, Golomb, Hodgkin's and non-Hodgkin's lymphomas,
      pp. 193–199 (Grune & Stratton, New York 1980).
12    Coller, B.S.; Chabner, B.A.; Gralnick, H.R.: Frequencies and patterns of bone
      marrow involvement in the non-Hodgkin's lymphomas: observation on the value of
      bilateral biopsies. Am. J. Hematol. 3: 105–119 (1979).
13    Come, S.E.; Chabner, B.A.: Staging in non-Hodgkin's lymphoma: approach, results
      and relationship to histopathology; in Canellos, Clinics in haematology, vol. 8,
      pp. 645–656 (Saunders, Philadelphia 1979).
14    Damber, L.; Lenner, P.; Lundgren, E.: The impact of growth pattern on survival in
      non-Hodgkin's lymphomas classified according to Lukes and Collins. Path. Res.
      Pract. 174: 42–52 (1982).
15    Dee, J.W.; Valdivieso, M.; Drewinki, B.: Comparison of the efficacies of closed
      trephine needle biopsy, aspirated paraffin-embedded clot section, and smear
      preparation in the diagnosis of bone-marrow involvement by lymphoma. Am. J. clin.
      Path. 65: 183–194 (1976).
16    Foucar, K.; McKenna, R.W.; Frizzera, G.; Brunning, R.D.: Incidence and patterns of
      bone marrow and blood involvement by lymphoma in relationship to the
      Lukes-Collins classification. Blood 54: 1417–1422 (1979).
17    Georgii, A.: Classification of non-Hodgkin's lymphomas from biopsies of the bone
      marrow with special emphasis to their spread; in Growther, Leukemia and
      non-Hodgkin's lymphoma, pp. 179–188 (Pergamon Press, Oxford 1979).
18    Glimelius, B.; Hagberg, H.; Sundström, C.: Morphological classification of
      non-Hodgkin's malignant lymphoma. II. Comparison between Rappaport's
      classification and the Kiel classification. Scand. J. Haematol. 30: 13–24 (1983).
19    Hashimoto, M.; Masanori, H.; Tsukasa, S.: Lymphoid nodules in human bone
      marrow. Acta path. jap. 7: 33–52 (1957).
20    Lennert, K.; Collins, R.D.; Lukes, R.J.: Concordance of the Kiel and Lukes-Collins
      classification of non-Hodgkin's lymphomas. Histopathology 7: 549–559 (1983).
21    Lennert, K.; Mohri, N.; Stein, H.; Kaiserling, E.: The histopathology of malignant
      lymphoma. Br. J. Haemat. 31: suppl., pp. 193–203 (1975).
22    Lennert, K.; Stein, H.: Histopathologie der Non-Hodgkin-Lymphome (nach der Kiel-
      Klassifikation) (Springer, Berlin 1981).
23    Lipshutz, M.D.; Mir, R.; Rai, K.R.; Sawitzky, A.: Bone marrow biopsy and clinical
      staging in chronic lymphocytic leukemia. Cancer 46: 1422–1427 (1980).
24    Lukes, R.J.; Collins, R.D.: New approaches to the classification of the lymphomata.
      Br. J. Cancer 31: suppl. 2, pp. 1–28 (1975).
25    Magrath, I.T.: Lymphocyte differentiation: an essential basis for the comprehension
      of lymphoid neoplasia. J. nat. Cancer Inst. 67: 501–514 (1981).
26    Natwani, B.N.: A critical analysis of the classification of non-Hodgkin's lymphomas.
      Cancer 44: 347–384 (1979).
27    Ralfkiaer, E.; Geisler, C.; Hansen, M.M.; Hou-Jensen, K.: Nuclear clefts in chronic
      lymphocytic leukaemia. A light microscopic and ultrastructural study of a new prog-
      nostic parameter. Scand. J. Haematol. 30: 5–12 (1983).

28 Rappaport, H.: Tumors of the hematopoietic system; in Atlas of tumor pathology, section 3, vol. 8 (Armed Forces Institute of Pathology, Washington 1966).

29 Rilke, F.; Pilotti, S.; Carbone, A.; Lombardi, L.: Morphology of lymphatic cells and of their derived tumours. J. clin. Path. *31:* 1009–1056 (1978).

30 Rosenberg, S.A.: Bone marrow involvement in the non-Hodgkin's lymphomata. Br. J. Cancer *31:* suppl. II, pp. 261–264 (1975).

31 Rosenberg, S.A.: Validity of the Ann Arbor staging classification for the non-Hodgkin's lymphomas. Cancer Treatm. Rep. *61:* 1023–1027 (1977).

32 Rozman, C.; Hernandez-Nieto, L.; Montserrat, E.; Brugues, R.: Prognostic significance of bone marrow patterns in chronic lymphocytic leukaemia. Br. J. Haemat. *47:* 529–537 (1981).

33 Rywlin, A.M.; Ortega, R.S.; Dominguez, C.J.: Lymphoid nodules of the bone marrow: normal and abnormal. Blood *43:* 389–400 (1974).

34 Sousa, M. de: Lymphocyte circulation: experimental and clinical aspects (Wiley, Chichester 1981).

35 Wright, D.H.: The identification and classification of non-Hodgkin's lymphoma: a review. Diagnostic Histopathology *5:* 73–111 (1982).

# 8  Hodgkin's Disease (HD)

## Survey of the Literature

In spite of recent advances in histologic diagnosis, in clinical staging and in treatment of patients in HD, the neoplastic cell clone specific for this disease has not been identified [11, 12, 23, 25]. The neoplastic tissue is composed of a variable number of morphologically and cytogenetically abnormal cells (Reed-Sternberg cells and their mononuclear counterparts) together with morphologically normal lymphocytes, eosinophils and mast cells [13]. The minimal requirement for the pathologic diagnosis of HD is the presence of characteristic giant cells of the Reed-Sternberg (RS) type in an appropriate histologic setting [13]. The Rye histopathologic classification into four subgroups – lymphocyte predominance (LP), nodular sclerosis (NS), mixed cellularity (MC) and lymphocyte depletion (LD) – was an important contribution to the prognostic evaluation of HD. Subsequently, accurate assessment of the extent of disease became mandatory when it was recognized that HD has a contiguous spread and therefore might be cured by radiotherapy to the involved site. since one of the criteria for systemic dissemination is involvement of the bone marrow, a bone biopsy is now an integral part of the investigation of patients at first presentation [3, 24]. Moreover, a sequential biopsy should be performed in all HD patients with advanced lymph node enlargement or in those who have pancytopenia of uncertain etiology, elevated serum alkaline phosphatase, bone scan abnormalities or systemic symptoms [14, 19]. The experience accumulated over the past decade has shown that adequate bone biopsies not only provide information on whether or not there is involvement, but also on the state of the non-involved marrow [1, 2, 4, 8, 27].

## Own Observations

A total of 661 patients with HD was investigated. The follow-up period ranged from 1 to 10 years, with a median of 3 years. In 491 cases, bone marrow biopsy was performed as part of the initial investigation, the remaining 170 patients had already received specific therapy and the biopsies were taken for restaging. In 641 patients the initial diagnosis of HD was made by histologic examination of lymph nodes, 20 patients were initially diagnosed by extranodal histology. In 5 cases the bone marrow remained the only documented site of HD, in spite of intensive investigation [9, 26]. Once the diagnosis was established, therapy was instituted according to the stage of the disease.

### Definition and Incidence of Bone Marrow Involvement

Identification of RS cells within granulomatous tissue is required for initial diagnosis (fig. 68), but when HD has already been documented elsewhere, atypical mononuclear cells within an appropriate setting plus lymphocytic infiltration may be taken as evidence of involvement (fig. 70). Biopsies with small epithelioid-cell granulomas or with foci of fibrosis or lymphoid nodules without mononuclear cells were grouped as 'negative' (fig. 72).

Bone marrow involvement was found in 14% of all the 661 patients investigated. At the time of initial diagnosis, the bone marrow was involved in 10% of the 491 untreated patients. In 11 cases the initial histologic diagnosis of HD was based on bone marrow histology. The incidence of positive bone marrow biopsies was strikingly different when the patients were grouped according to histologic classification or clinical stages, as shown in table XIV.

Table XIV. Frequency of bone marrow involvement in HD (491 pretreatment patients)

|  | Patients | Positive bone marrow biopsies, % |
|---|---|---|
| *Clinical stage* | | |
| I | 168 | 1 |
| II | 212 | 2 |
| III | 72 | 25 |
| IV | 28 | 45 |
| *Lymph node histology* | | |
| LP | 53 | 8 |
| NS | 197 | 4 |
| MC | 173 | 9 |
| LD | 47 | 22 |
| HD, total | 491 | 10 |

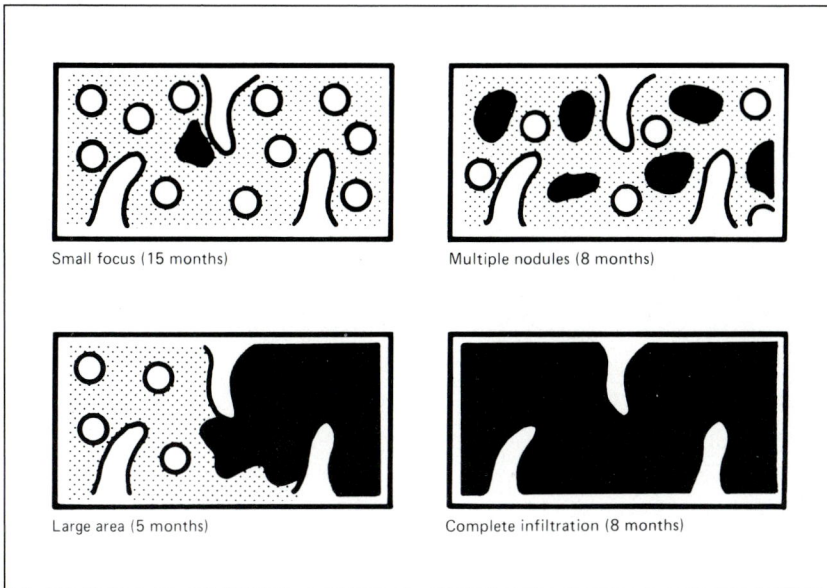

Fig. 65. Patterns of HD in the bone marrow histology and their prognostic relevance (median survival time).

### Histologic Features of Bone Marrow Manifestation

Positive biopsies revealed four growth patterns (fig. 65): (1) a single, small focus, with a predominantly paratrabecular location, (2) multiple nodules of 1–4 mm in diameter, dispersed throughout the bone marrow cavities, (3) a large, solitary focus occupying more than one marrow space, usually accompanied by osteolytic or osteosclerotic reactions, and (4) complete replacement of the marrow tissue. RS cells were identified in 62% and mononuclear Hodgkin cells in 95% of the positive biopsies.

### Identification of Prognostic Factors in Bone Marrow Histology

Seven histologic parameters were analyzed to test their prognostic relevance. The most significant prognostic factor proved to be the demonstration of bone marrow involvement. Pretreatment patients with a positive bone marrow biopsy had significantly shorter survival times than those with a negative biopsy (fig. 66, tables XV, XVI).

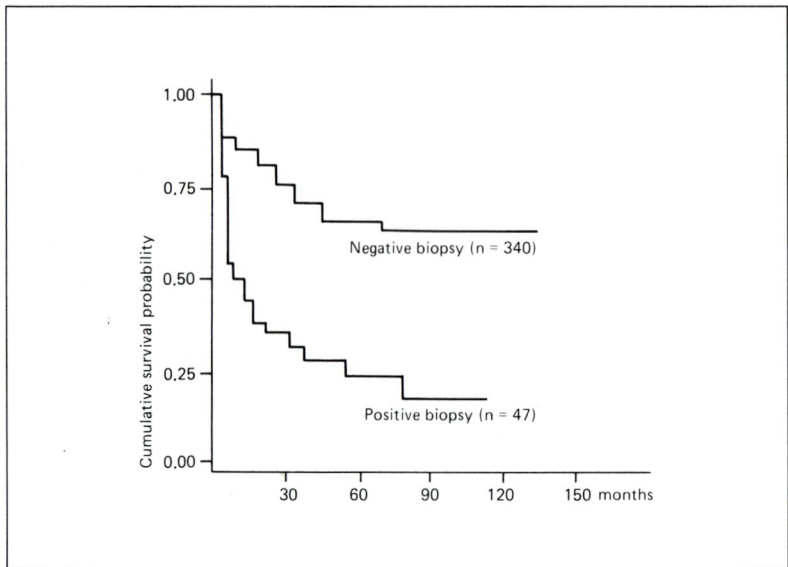

**Fig. 66.** Predictive value of bone marrow histology in HD; grouping variable is 'bone marrow involvement'.

**Table XV.** Prognostic factors of HD in the bone marrow biopsy

| Histologic criteria | Patients | Median survival months | Breslow, Mantel-Cox p values |
|---|---|---|---|
| Lymphocytes | | | 0.0423 |
| Few | 50 | 5 | 0.0321 |
| Many | 19 | 52 | |
| Reed-Sternberg cells | | | 0.1211 |
| Low degree | 31 | 13 | 0.3707 |
| High degree | 40 | 5 | |
| Infiltration | | | 0.2749 |
| < 30 vol% | 25 | 9 | 0.3249 |
| ≥ 30 vol% | 56 | 5 | |
| Bone remodelling | | | 0.2206 |
| Normal | 39 | 9 | 0.2954 |
| Osteoblastic | 21 | 6 | |
| Osteoclastic | 11 | 4 | |

**Table XVI.** Histologic classification of HD and other granulomatous disorders in the bone marrow – 143 patients

| | HD lymphocyte depletion | HD lymphocyte predominance | Systemic mastocytosis | Angioimmunoblastic 'myelopathy' |
|---|---|---|---|---|
| Patients | 50 | 19 | 62 | 12 |
| Male/female | 2.1 | 3.3 | 1.4 | 0.7 |
| Age, median, years | 47 | 39 | 48 | 50 |
| Osteoporosis (X ray), % | 10 | 13 | 18 | 0 |
| Osteolysis (X ray), % | 6 | 4 | 25 | 0 |
| Osteosclerosis (X ray), % | 0 | 8 | 28 | 0 |
| Lymphomas, % | 65 | 61 | 0 | 67 |
| Splenomegaly, % | 17 | 39 | 12 | 80 |
| Anaemia (Hb < 10 g/dl), % | 36 | 25 | 8 | 40 |
| Leukopenia (<4 $\times$ 10$^9$/l), % | 28 | 12 | 10 | 81 |
| Thrombopenia (<200 $\times$ 10$^9$/l), % | 38 | 29 | 62 | 81 |
| ESR, mm/h | 86 (40) | 58 (42) | 16 (20) | 83 (46) |
| Infiltration, vol% | 38 (22) | 35 (24) | 12 (10) | 40 (17) |
| Haematopoietic tissue, vol% | 19 (14) | 17 (18) | 33 (14) | 17 (10) |
| Fatty tissue, vol% | 10 (10) | 9 (10) | 20 (12) | 14 (10) |
| Sinusoids, vol% | 2 (2) | 3 (2) | 5 (4) | 2 (1) |
| Trabecular bone, vol% | 23 (5) | 25 (5) | 26 (8) | 24 (5) |
| Growth pattern | | | | |
| Solitary small focus, % | 7 | 19 | 25 | 0 |
| Confluent foci, % | 24 | 81 | 55 | 100 |
| Complete infiltration, % | 69 | 0 | 20 | 0 |

Numbers in parentheses = standard deviations.

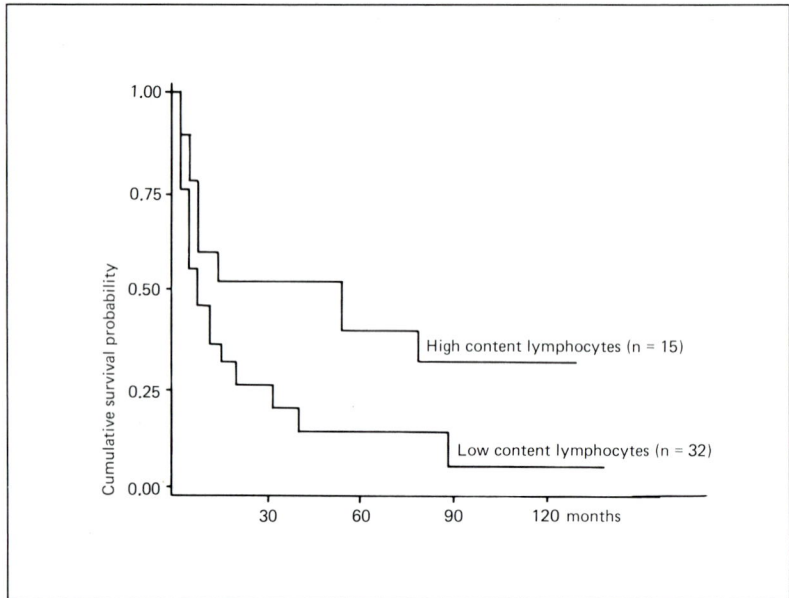

**Fig. 67.** Predictive value of bone marrow biopsy in HD with positive biopsies; grouping variable is 'degree of lymphocytic infiltration'.

Data of 47 pretreatment patients with positive biopsies were available for survival statistics. The following histologic variables were analyzed to test their suitability as criteria for classification of bone marrow manifestations in HD: quantity of lymphogranulomatous tissue (vol%), degree of lymphocytic infiltration, presence of RS cells, type of osseous remodelling and of fibrosis, degree of eosinophilic reactions and of oedema. Of all these parameters only the degree of lymphocytic infiltration proved to be a reliable predictive factor. Patients with a low content of lymphocytes (32 cases) had a much shorter life expectancy than those 15 cases with a high content (fig. 67, 68). The comparison of the 47 pre- and the 26 posttreatment patients with positive biopsies revealed no differences in survival (median survivals of 8 and 7 months, respectively). Further 4 cases of HD were characterized by a high content of epithelioid cells in the lymphogranulomatous tissue (fig. 69).

Data of 332 pretreatment patients with negative biopsies were also analyzed. Though the 10 patients with epithelioid-cell granulomas (fig. 71) in the bone marrow are too few for a reliable statistic analysis, they had a very favourable prognosis with a long, smouldering course (fig. 72). Long survival times were also found in the patients with atrophic changes of the bone marrow, but there was a more unfavourable course in the late part of the cumulative survival curve. Patients with a leukaemoid reaction had the worst prognosis (fig. 72).

*Other Lesions of Undetermined Etiology*

*Systemic mastocytosis (SM)* is a very rare disorder, usually diagnosed by skin biopsy [10, 17, 18, 28], and unless the pathologist is familiar with its typical histology, misinterpretation often occurs. We investigated bone marrow biopsies from 78 adult patients with established SM, and bone marrow involvement was evident in 80% of the cases (prospective study, in collaboration with *H.G. Rohner,* St. Barbara Hospital, Gladbeck, FRG). The characteristic histologic lesion was the mast cell granuloma with predominantly prominent paratrabecular and paravascular arrangement. In advanced cases, the granulomas had coalesced and occupied large areas or even completely replaced the haematopoietic tissues and had evoked striking osseous reactions, both lytic and sclerotic. The granulomatous tissue consisted of a central area of spindle-shaped mast cells, lymphocytes and small vessels, with a rim of plasma cells, eosinophils and, in some cases, of 'sea-blue' histiocytes. Survival statistics documented a very favourable life expectancy: within a follow-up period of 4 years only 3 of 25 patients with SM have died. The indolent course as well as the granulomatous features in SM suggest an immunologic, non-neoplastic pathogenesis, favouring the designation of mast cell granulomatosis. Malignant (immature) types of systemic mastocytosis were observed in only 4 cases.

*Angioimmunoblastic lymphadenopathy (AILD)* is also considered to be a systemic disorder of undetermined biology which frequently involves the bone marrow [7, 16, 21, 22]. In our material of 20 cases with AILD, diagnosed by the lymph node biopsy, bone marrow involvement was found in 12 cases. The typical growth pattern in the bone marrow was multifocal or partly confluent, and comparable with those patterns described in HD and SM. The cellular composition reflects primarily that of the involved lymph nodes: a heterogenous population of lymphocytes, plasma cells, histiocytes and immunoblasts within a network of reticulin fibres and arborising capillaries (fig. 73). Patients with AILD and bone marrow manifestations had a relatively short life expectancy: only 5 of 12 patients survived a follow-up period of 4 years.

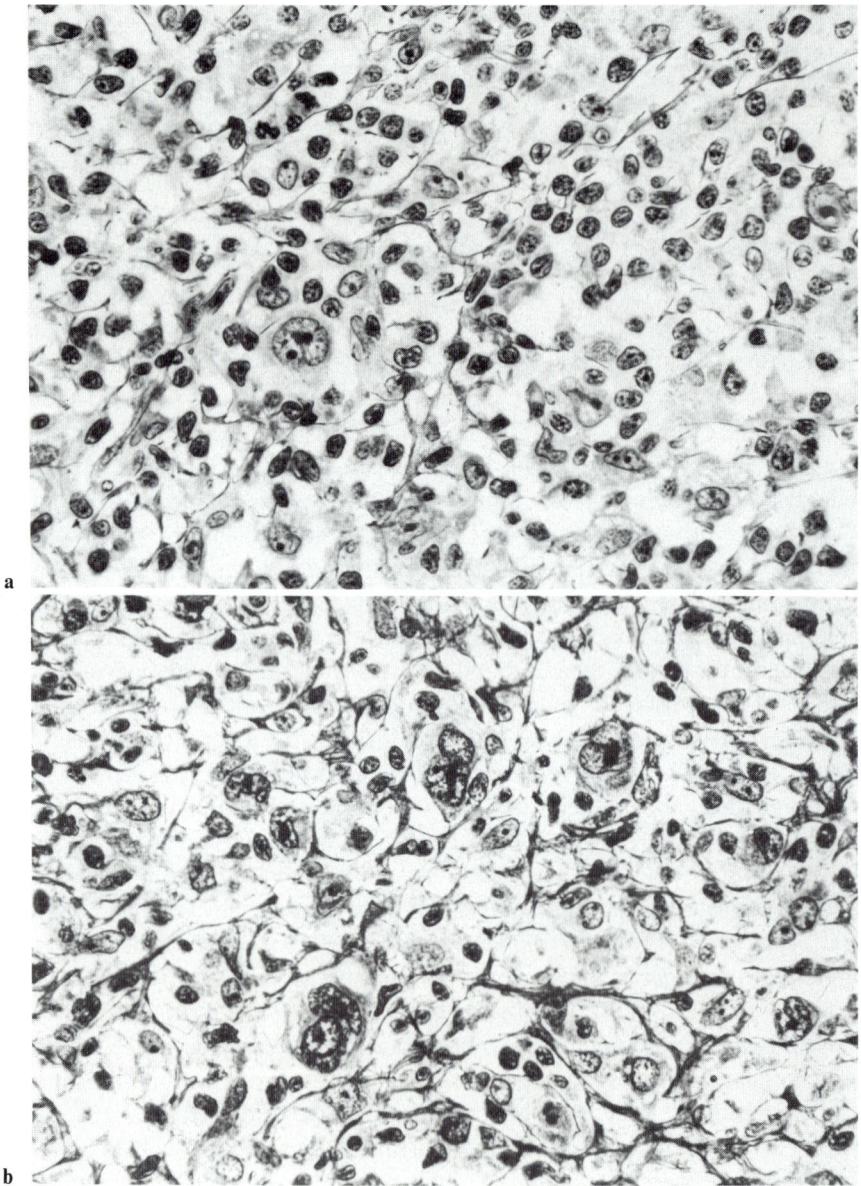

**Fig. 68.** Histologic types of HD in the bone marrow biopsy. Gomori. ✕ 250. **a** Lymphogranulomatous tissue with high content of lymphocytes. **b** Lymphogranulomatous tissue with low content of lymphocytes.

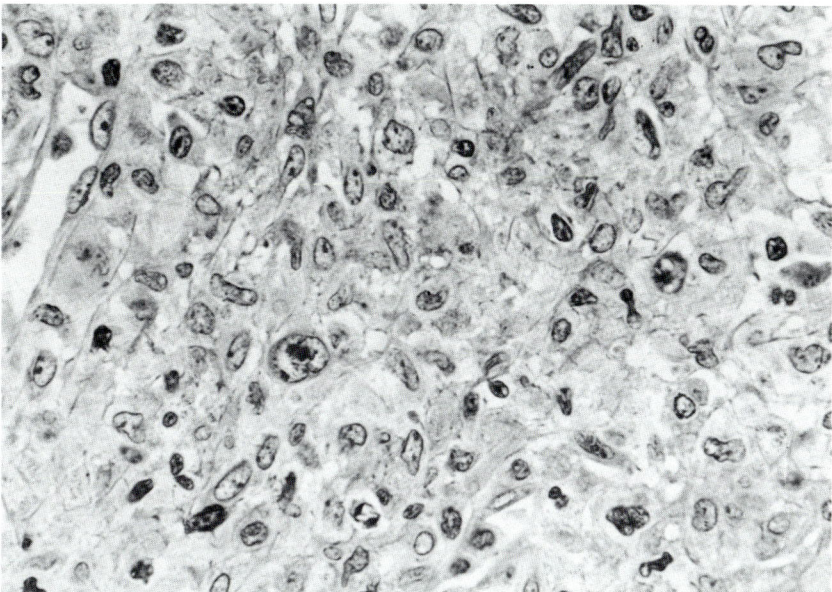

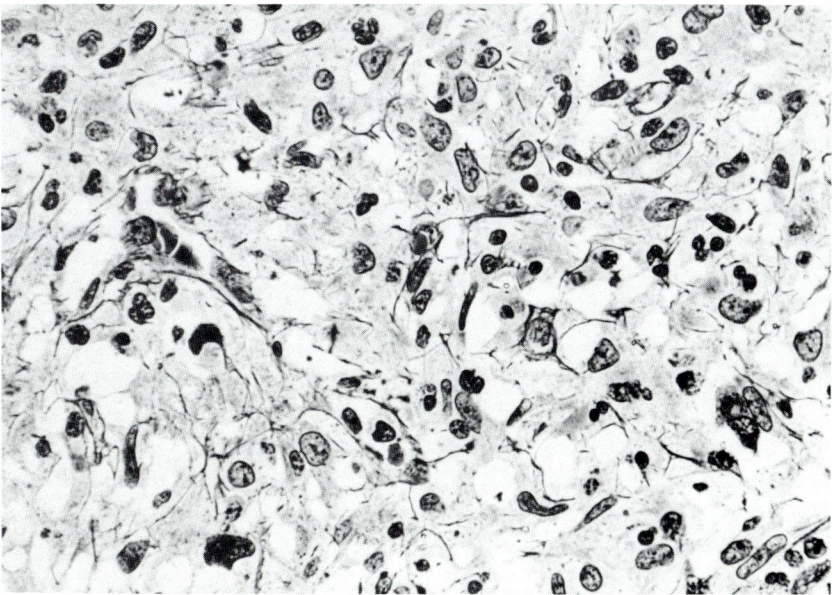

**Fig. 69.** Lymphogranulomatous tissue with high content of epithelioid cells. Gomori. × 400.

**Fig. 70.** Granulomatous tissue with atypical mononuclear cells and lymphocytes in bone marrow histology. Diagnosis of HD already established by lymph node histology. Gomori. × 400.

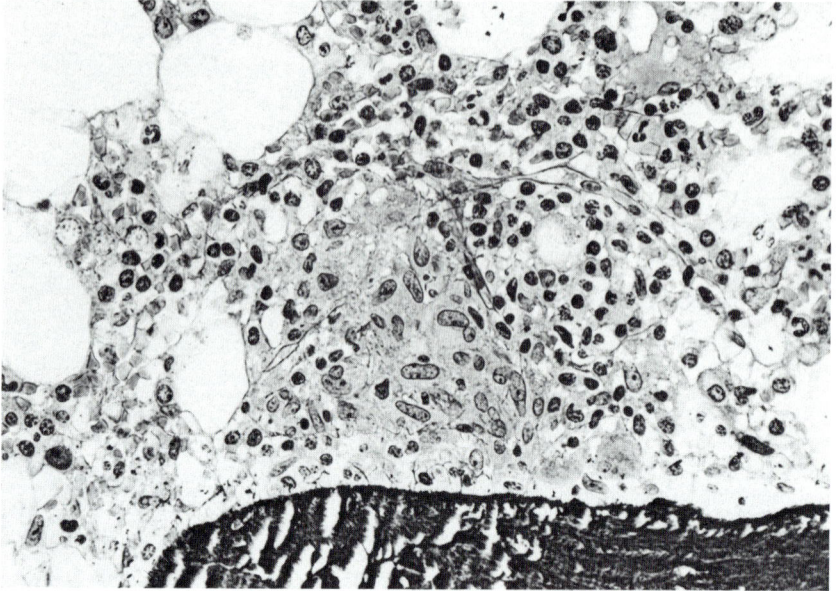

**Fig. 71.** Epithelioid-cell granuloma in the bone marrow histology in HD. Gomori. × 100.

## Implications for Medical Practice

This study of bone marrow biopsies in HD has shown an overall incidence of 10% in untreated patients, while the results of previous series have ranged from 2 to 32% [5, 6, 15]. Various factors may influence the rate of detection: (1) selection of patients, (2) biopsy techniques and histologic preparation, and (3) differences in the interpretation of the histologic findings. It has previously been shown that a large single or two bilateral, smaller biopsies are about equally effective [1, 2]. The probability of bone marrow involvement was significantly higher in the presence of B symptoms, pancytopenia, hepatomegaly or an elevated serum alkaline phosphatase [19]. Also patients with lymphocytic depletion type in the lymph node histology as well as in clinical stages III and IV had a much higher risk of bone marrow spread, in contrast to a very low risk in the NS type.

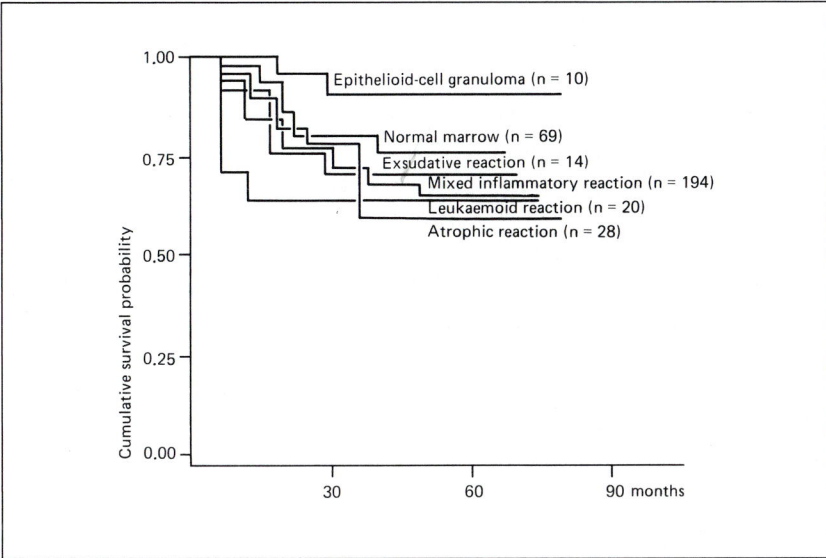

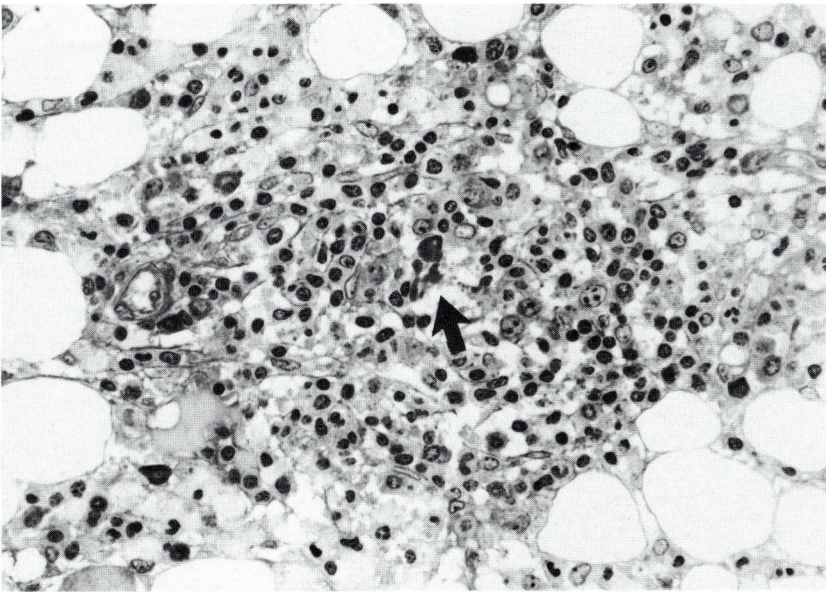

**Fig. 72.** Predictive value of bone marrow biopsy in HD with negative biopsies; grouping variable is 'type of non-specific reaction'.

**Fig. 73.** Angioimmunoblastic 'myelopathy' with high content of capillaries and interstitial PAS-positive deposits (arrow). Giemsa. × 400.

HD manifestations in the bone marrow can be classified into those with a high content of lymphocytes and a more favourable prognosis, and those with a low content of lymphocytes and a less favourable prognosis. This grouping of lymphogranulomatous tissue in the bone marrow is simple, reproducible and prognostically significant.

Non-caseating epithelioid-cell granulomas in HD have been found in lymph nodes, spleen and bone marrow, in about 15% of the patients [20]. As the presence of these granulomas was never associated with specific lesions and correlated with a strikingly favourable prognosis, they might well be considered as morphologic expressions of a host response against the disease.

Three conclusions of prognostic significance may be drawn from these results: that bone marrow involvement is already present in 10% of all patients with HD at first presentation, that the bone marrow lesions are classifiable, and that in 80% of cases without involvement the bone marrow shows reactive changes which have prognostic significance.

## References

1   Bartl, R.; Burkhardt, R.; Lengsfeld, H.; Huhn, D.: Die Bedeutung der histologischen Knochenmarksbeurteilung bei Morbus Hodgkin. Klin. Wschr. *54:* 1061–1075 (1976).
2   Bartl, R.; Frisch, B.; Burkhardt, R.; Huhn, D.; Pappenberger, R.: Assessment of bone marrow histology in Hodgkin's disease: correlation with clinical factors. Br. J. Haemat. *51:* 345–360 (1982).
3   Brunning, R.D.; McKenna, R.W.: Bone marrow manifestations of malignant lymphoma and lymphoma-like conditions; in Sommers, Rosen, Pathology annual 1979, part I, pp. 1–59 (Appleton-Century-Crofts, New York 1979).
4   Burkhardt, R.; Zettl, R.; Bartl, R.: Significance of non-specific changes of the bone marrow tissues from the bioptic viewpoint. Biblthca haemat., vol. 45, pp. 38–49 (Karger, Basel 1978).
5   Chabner, B.A.; Gralnick, H.R.; Myers, C.E.; Vita, V.T. de: Bone marrow involvement in Hodgkin's disease (HD): pathology and clinical implications. Ann. intern. Med. *78:* 824 (1973).
6   Colby, T.V.; Hoppe, R.T.; Warnke, R.A.: Hodgkin's disease at autopsy: 1972–1977. Cancer, N.Y. *47:* 1852–1862 (1981).
7   Ershlev, W.B.; Moore, A.L.; Stanley, L.B.; Tindle, B.H.: Immunoblastic lymphadenopathy: failure of rather than lack of immunoregulation. J. Med. *14:* 81–94 (1983).
8   Georgii, A.; Vykoupil, K.F.: Unspecific mesenchymal reaction in bone marrow in patients with Hodgkin's disease; in Musshoff, Diagnosis and therapy of malignant lymphoma, pp. 39–43 (Springer, Berlin 1970).

9  Heider, K.: Über Knochengranulomatose mit besonderer Berücksichtigung der primären Erscheinungsformen. Z. klin. Med. *136:* 240–257 (1936).

10  Horny, H.P.; Parwaresch, M.R.; Lennert, K.: Klinisches Bild und Prognose generalisierter Mastozytosen. Klin. Wschr. *61:* 785–793 (1983).

11  Kaplan, H.S.: Hodgkin's disease: unfolding concepts concerning its nature, management and prognosis. Cancer *45:* 2439–2474 (1980).

12  Long, J.C.: The immunopathology of Hodgkin's disease; in Canellos, Clinics in haematology, vol. 8, pp. 531–566 (Saunders, London 1979).

13  Lukes, R.J.: Criteria for involvement of lymph node, bone marrow, spleen and liver in Hodgkin's disease. Cancer Res. *31:* 1755–1769 (1971).

14  Myers, C.E.; Chabner, B.A.; Vita, V.T. de; Gralnick, H.R.: Bone marrow involvement in Hodgkin's disease: pathology and response to MOPP chemotherapy. Blood *44:* 197–204 (1974).

15  O'Carroll, D.I.; McKenna, R.W.; Brunning, R.D.: Bone marrow manifestations of Hodgkin's disease. Cancer, N.Y. *38:* 1717–1728 (1976).

16  Pangalis, G.A.; Moran, E.M.; Rappaport, H.: Blood and bone marrow findings in angioimmunoblastic lymphadenopathy. Blood *51:* 71–83 (1978).

17  Rohner, H.G.; Bartl, R.; Klingmüller, G.; Kreysel, H.W.; Geisler, L.S.: Die Mastozytose – eine Krankheit mit häufiger Systemisierung. Therapiewoche *30:* 6773–6779 (1980).

18  Rohner, H.G.; Bartl, R.; Koischwitz, D.; Rodermund, O.-E.: Haut- und Knochenbefunde bei der Mastozytose. Radiologe *22:* 545–552 (1982).

19  Rosenberg, S.A.: Hodgkin's disease of the bone marrow. Cancer Res. *31:* 1733–1736 (1971).

20  Sacks, E.L.; Donaldson, S.S.; Gordon, J.; Dorfman, R.F.: Epithelioid granulomas associated with Hodgkin's disease. Clinical correlations in 55 previously untreated patients. Cancer, N.Y. *41:* 562–567 (1978).

21  Schauer, P.D.; Straus, D.J.; Bagley, C.M., et al.: Angioimmunoblastic lymphadenopathy: clinical spectrum of disease. Cancer *48:* 2493–2498 (1981).

22  Schnaidt, U.; Vykoupil, K.F.; Thiele, J.; Georgii, A.: Angioimmunoblastic lymphadenopathy. Histopathology of bone marrow involvement. Virchows Arch. Abt. A Path. Anat. *389:* 369–380 (1980).

23  Stuart, A.E.: Pathogenesis of Hodgkin's disease. J. Path. *12:* 239–254 (1978).

24  Sutcliffe, S.B.J.; Timothy, A.R.; Lister, T.A.: Staging in Hodgkin's disease; in Canellos, Clinics in haematology, vol. 8, pp. 593–609 (Saunders, Philadelphia 1979).

25  Taylor, C.R.: Immunopathology of Hodgkin's disease; in van den Tweel et al., Malignant lymphoproliferative diseases, pp. 399–416 (Leiden University Press, Leiden 1980).

26  Uehlinger, E.: Über Knochenlymphogranulomatose. Virchows Arch. path. Anat. Physiol. *288:* 36–118 (1933).

27  Velde, J. te; Ottolander, J.G. den; Spaander, P.J.; Berg, C. van den; Hartgrink-Groeneveld, C.A.: The bone marrow in Hodgkin's disease: the non-involved marrow. Histopathology *2:* 31–46 (1978).

28  Webb, T.A.; Li, C.Y.; Yam, L.T.: Systemic mast cell disease: a clinical and hematopathologic study of 26 cases. Cancer *49:* 927–938 (1982).

# 9 Haematologic Malignancies (HM) in the Bone Marrow

## A Summary of Our Observations

### Survey of the Literature

The question as to whether neoplasias arise from single cells or have a multicellular origin is of particular importance because of its therapeutic consequences. Most carcinomas appear to have a unicentric origin, with subsequent dissemination by various processes, some of which can be understood on a mechanical basis [1, 3, 14]. Nevertheless, it is difficult to exclude a multicentric origin for epithelial tumours, since in these cases it is wellnigh impossible to separate multicentric tumours from unicentric ones with metastases [3]. The situation is completely different in haematologic neoplasias. Very rarely do isolated tumours occur which then metastasize *(blastomas)*. Occasionally there may be multicentric tumours *(blastomatoses)* as such, however, the most frequently encountered haematologic malignancies are the *blastoses* which spread throughout the blood-forming organs and then spill over into the blood [6]. Transitions between multicentric aleukaemic and leukaemic variants were previously listed under the heading of systemic HM [3].

HM are assigned either to the *myeloid* or the *lymphoid* systems. Malignancies previously designated as reticuloses are now thought to arise from myeloid or lymphoid precursors [8]: the 'small cell reticulosis' as well as most cases of 'reticular sarcomas' are regarded as lymphomas [7], and 'mast cell reticulosis' is claimed to belong to the monocytic cell line and therefore has a myeloid origin [8]. The neoplastic nature and cellular origin of Hodgkin's disease (lymphogranulomatosis) has still not been elucidated but because of its lymphoma-like nature it has traditionally been assigned to the group of the lymphoid neoplasias [9].

All haematologic neoplasias have in common their derivation from pluripotent stem cells. Recent investigations have shown that haematologic neoplasias have a monoclonal origin, at least the ones that have so far been investigated [5, 10, 11]. The subsequent histologic structure and the clinical picture are determined by the capacity for proliferation and differentiation of the pathologic clone [2, 4, 10, 12, 13]. Based on this concept the HM were separated into several large groups and the haematologic and clinical findings as well as the histomorphology were utilized to determine criteria of prognostic significance.

## Summary of Our Observations

### Bone Marrow Involvement in HM

The diagnosis of *MPD* in the bone marrow biopsy usually presented no problems, though in a few cases of PV the proliferative activity was very low and follow-up studies were necessary to confirm the diagnosis.

Likewise, in a few cases of *AL* the number of blast cells was so small that only a combined assessment of histology, cytology and cytochemistry enabled a definite diagnosis to be made.

In the group of the *plasma cell neoplasms,* a systemic manifestation with positive bone marrow biopsies was found in 80%, confirming the diagnosis of *MM.* In further 5% of the cases the plasmacellular infiltration was so small that diagnosis of MM was only possible by immunohistologic demonstration of monoclonal plasma cells. Plasmablastic sarcomas with metastatic spread in the bone marrow were found in the biopsies in another 5%. The last 10% of the cases with clinical evidence of plasmacytoma showed negative bone marrow biopsies; these patients had solitary or at least paucifocal plasmacytomas.

In the heterogenous *NHL,* the systemic groups with a leukaemic blood picture (e.g. CLL) always showed bone marrow involvement in large-scale biopsies. In the 'aleukaemic' subgroups (e.g. immunocytoma), the incidence of bone marrow involvement was 80%. The groups with primarily regional manifestations (e.g. centroblastic/centrocytic lymphoma) and with sarcomatous growth patterns (e.g. immunoblastic sarcoma) had positive bone marrow biopsies in about 25% of the cases.

The lowest incidence (10%) at the time of first presentation was found in *HD.* The LD type in the lymph node histology correlated with a significantly higher incidence of bone marrow involvement than the NS type (22 and 4%, respectively).

**Table XVII.** Prognostic factors of HM in the bone marrow biopsy

| Criteria | Patients | Median survival months | Breslow, Mantel-Cox p values |
|---|---|---|---|
| Cell maturity | | | 0.0001 |
|   Mature | 710 | 48 | 0.0001 |
|   Immature | 170 | 4 | |
| Proliferative cell line | | | 0.0001 |
|   Erythrocytic | 206 | 82 | 0.0001 |
|   Megakaryocytic | 64 | 51 | |
|   Granulocytic | 207 | 12 | |
|   Monocytic | 17 | 4 | |
|   Lymphocytic | 427 | 26 | |
|   Plasmacytic | 245 | 26 | |
| Mitotic activity | | | 0.0001 |
|   Low | 163 | 46 | 0.0001 |
|   Intermediate | 452 | 17 | |
|   High | 110 | 6 | |
| Infiltration | | | 0.0001 |
|   < 20 vol% | 198 | 47 | 0.0002 |
|   20–50 vol% | 179 | 15 | |
|   > 50 vol% | 228 | 12 | |
| Fatty tissue | | | 0.0226 |
|   < 5 vol% | 663 | 23 | 0.0050 |
|   5–25 vol% | 342 | 38 | |
|   > 25 vol% | 100 | 48 | |
| Degree of fibrosis | | | 0.1250 |
|   Normal | 228 | 49 | 0.0169 |
|   Fine | 596 | 27 | |
|   Fine, partly coarse | 170 | 20 | |
|   Coarse | 62 | 45 | |
|   Coarse, woven bone | 51 | 50 | |
| Bone remodelling | | | 0.1207 |
|   Normal | 878 | 31 | 0.0538 |
|   Osteoblastic | 90 | 44 | |
|   Osteoblastic/osteoclastic | 69 | 26 | |
|   Osteoclastic | 70 | 15 | |
| Stromal reaction | | | 0.3142 |
|   Absent | 588 | 33 | 0.3502 |
|   Low | 158 | 24 | |
|   High | 239 | 27 | |

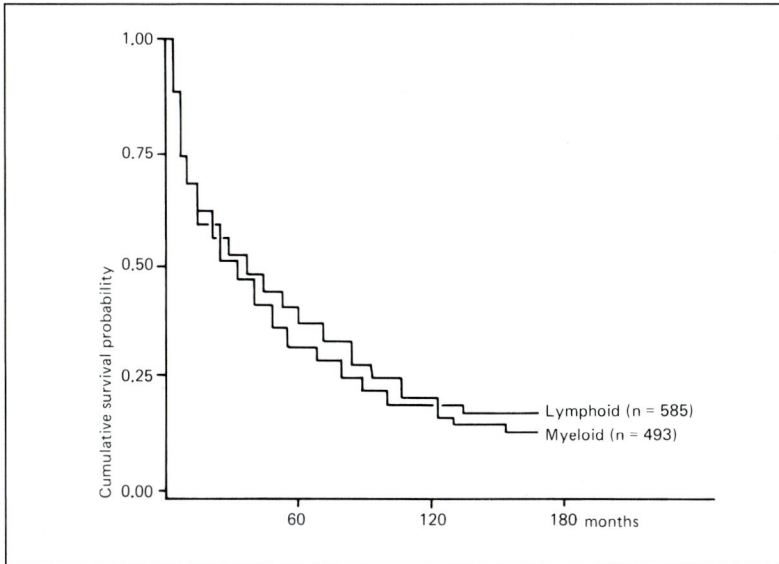

**Fig. 74.** Predictive value of bone marrow histology in HM; grouping variable is 'proliferative cell system'.

*Identification of Prognostic Factors in the Bone Marrow Histology*

1,184 untreated patients with haematologic neoplasias in the bone marrow were assigned to one group and statistically analyzed for prognostic factors. Six common clinical and 15 histologic parameters were investigated for their predictive value; these are listed in table XVII.

Males had significantly shorter survivals than females. Patients younger than 20 and older than 70 years showed a less favourable prognosis. When the malignancies were divided into a myeloid and a lymphoid group, the life tables of the patients in each group were almost identical (fig. 74). But when the clinical groups with bone marrow involvement were separately analyzed, significant differences in prognosis were observed (fig. 75).

The most significant and most reliable factor for prognostic evaluation proved to be the maturity of the proliferative cell system in the bone marrow histology. Patients with predominantly mature (non-nucleolated) cells had highly significant longer survival durations than those with predominantly immature (nucleolated) cells (fig. 76). When grouped according to the proliferating cell lines, patients with the erythroid cell line had the best, those with the granulopoietic line the worst prognosis (table XVIII, fig. 77).

**75**

**76**

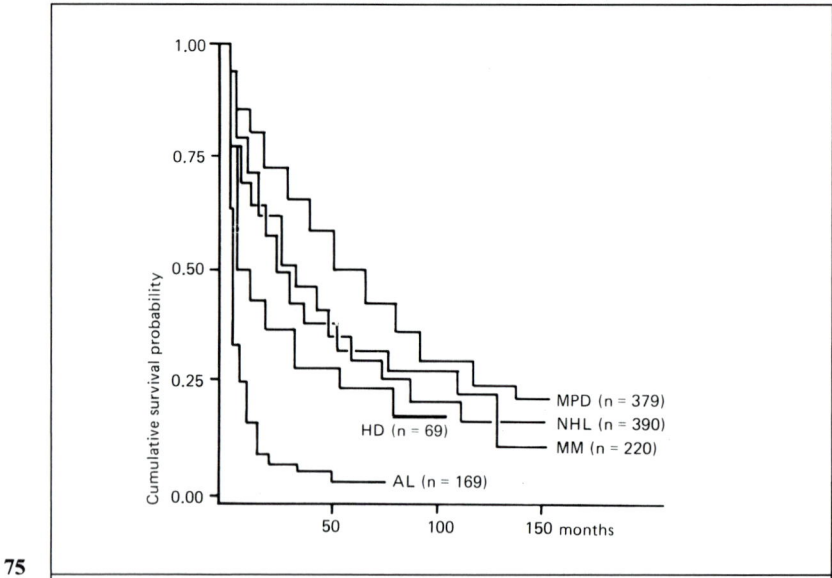

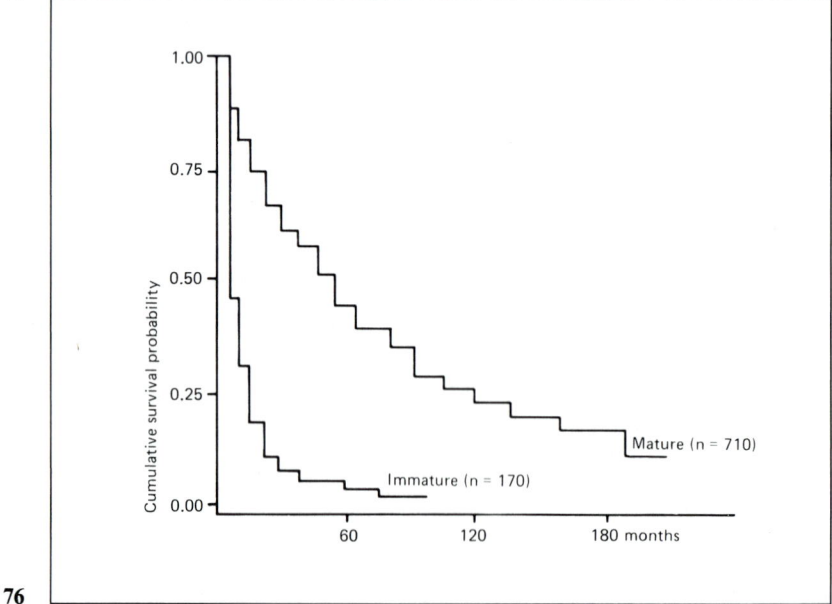

Fig. 75. Predictive value of bone marrow histology in HM; grouping variable is 'clinical entity'.

Fig. 76. Predictive value of bone marrow histology in HM; grouping variable is 'cell maturity'.

**Table XVIII.** Histologic classification of HM in the bone marrow biopsy

| Histologic type | Patients | Median survival (months) from time of | |
|---|---|---|---|
| | | initial biopsy | first symptom |
| Haematologic malignancies | 1,184 | 29 | 47 |
| Myeloid malignancies | 514 | 34 | 56 |
| Mature myeloid malignancies | 358 | 50 | 158 |
| Erythrocytic | 10 | 115 | 150 |
| Erythro-/granulocytic | 12 | 99 | 131 |
| Erythro-/megakaryocytic | 92 | 84 | 140 |
| Erythro-/megakaryo-/granulocytic | 77 | 79 | 158 |
| Megakaryocytic | 53 | 63 | 88 |
| Granulocytic | 52 | 18 | 40 |
| Granulo-/megakaryocytic | 62 | 27 | 37 |
| Immature myeloid malignancies | 156 | 4 | 14 |
| Myeloblastic | 63 | 3 | 11 |
| Myelomonocytic | 27 | 5 | 12 |
| Monoblastic | 17 | 3 | 12 |
| Promyelocytic | 23 | 3 | 15 |
| Erythroblastic | 15 | 2 | 9 |
| Megakaryoblastic | 11 | 4 | 20 |
| Lymphoid malignancies | 670 | 26 | 42 |
| Mature lymphoid malignancies | 514 | 35 | 54 |
| Lymphocytic | 132 | 41 | 64 |
| Hairy cell | 87 | 21 | 36 |
| Immunocytic | 90 | 44 | 72 |
| Centrocytic | 20 | 25 | 40 |
| Centroblastic/cytic | 17 | 50 | 60 |
| Plasmacytic | 149 | 32 | 41 |
| HD, lymphocyte predominance | 19 | 52 | 68 |
| Immature lymphoid malignancies | 156 | 7 | 16 |
| Lymphoblastic | 21 | 8 | 14 |
| Immunoblastic | 7 | 4 | 6 |
| Centroblastic | 7 | 5 | 9 |
| Plasmablastic | 71 | 8 | 19 |
| HD, lymphocyte depletion | 50 | 5 | 29 |

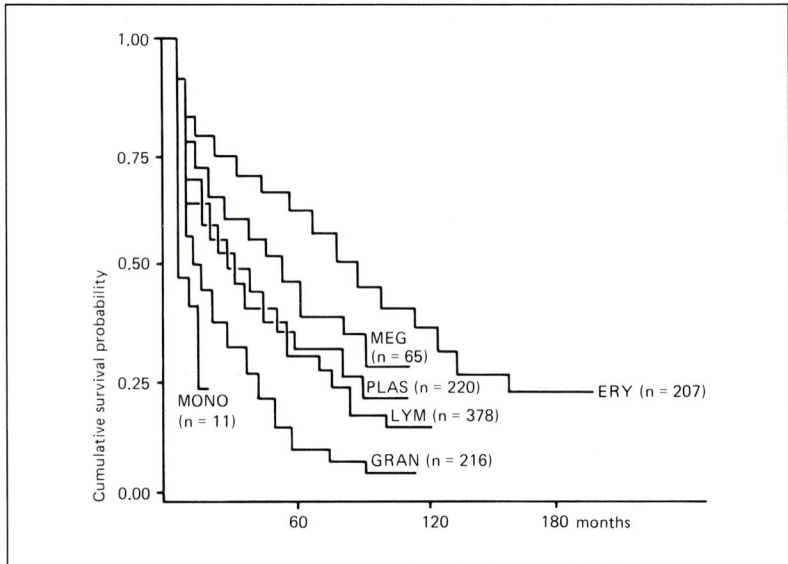

**Fig. 77.** Predictive value of bone marrow histology in HM; grouping variable is 'proliferative cell line'. ERY = Erythrocytic; MEG = megakaryocytic; GRAN = granulocytic; MONO = monocytic; PLAS = plasmacytic; LYM = lymphocytic.

The survival curves for the lymphocytic and plasmacytic lines were identical (26 months). Further cellular criteria of prognostic significance proved to be mitotic activity and cellular polymorphism. A nodular proliferation pattern in the bone marrow indicated a better prognosis than a diffuse pattern. Likewise, an increasing degree of neoplastic cell burden in the biopsy (vol%) correlated significantly with shorter survivals. Other histologic criteria such as stromal reactions, the degree of fatty tissue, fibrosis, vascularization, plasma cells, mast cells and osseous remodelling had some predictive value, but without statistical significance.

**Implications for Medical Practice**

In this study on HM in the bone marrow, four histologic elements proved to be of prognostic relevance (fig. 78): (1) the *proliferative cell system,* which represents the haematologic neoplasia; (2) the *proliferation pattern,* which describes the growth of the neoplasia; (3) the *tumour cell burden*

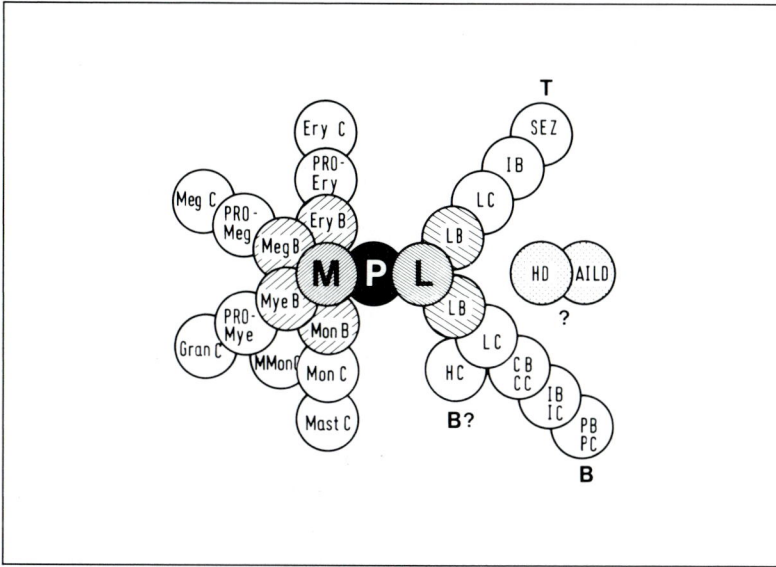

**Fig. 78.** Classification of haematologic malignancies according to the proliferative cell systems. P, M, L = Pluripotent, myeloid and lymphoid stem cells.

(vol%), which reflects the extent of the neoplasia, and (4) the *stromal reactions,* evoked by the neoplasia, which influence the progression of the disease.

These structural parameters in the bone marrow histology form the basis of a histologic classification and staging system for HM, proposed in this study:

(1) *MPD* were classified according to the proliferating haematopoietic cell line(s). The degree of fibrosis and of cell maturity were additional prognostic factors as well as reliable indicators for transformation or metamorphosis in MPD.

(2) *AL* were classified according to the proliferating cell type (cytologic, cytochemical and histologic criteria). Histologic parameters in the biopsy, such as degree of infiltration (vol%), quantity of fat cells (vol%), and of fibrosis, also proved to be of predictive value.

(3) *MM* was classified, analogous to NHL, according to plasma cell maturity into a plasmacytic (of low-grade malignancy) and a plasmablastic (of high-grade malignancy) cell type. The histomorphometric assessment of

plasma cell burden in the biopsy was used as a criterion for a histologic three-tier staging system.

(4) *NHL* in the bone marrow were classified according to the proliferating system, applying the Kiel nomenclature derived from lymph node histology. The various classes were subgrouped according to the different histotopographic growth patterns in the bone marrow. Primarily systemic, cumulative disorders were staged according to the volume of lymphoid infiltration in the biopsy (vol%).

(5) *HD* in the bone marrow was classified according to the degree of lymphocytic infiltration into a lymphocyte predominance and a lymphocyte depletion group. Non-specific changes in the bone marrow, including epithelioid-cell granulomas, are also of predictive value in HD.

In conclusion, bone marrow biopsy has proved its value, not only for diagnosis and prognosis, but also during subsequent treatment. The consequences of therapy – success or failure, and complications – may be quantitatively and qualitatively evaluated. Thus, in the bone marrow biopsy the clinician has a tool at his disposal which can supply valuable information on the diagnosis, prognosis and follow-up of patients with HM.

### References

1   Baldwin, R.W.: Secondary spread of cancer (Academic Press, London 1978).
2   Burkhardt, R.; Frisch, B.; Bartl, R.: Bone biopsy in haematological disorders. J. clin. Path. *35:* 257–284 (1982).
3   Eder, M.: Pathologie des Wachstums und der Differenzierung; in Lehrbuch der allgemeinen Pathologie und der pathologischen Anatomie, pp. 207–269 (Springer, Berlin 1977).
4   Frisch, B.; Bartl, R.; Burkhardt, R.: Bone marrow biopsy in clinical medicine: an overview. Haematologia *3:* 245–285 (1982).
5   Galton, D.A.G.: The chronic leukaemias; in Hoffbrand, Brain, Hirsh, Recent advances in haematology, vol. 2, pp. 219–242 (Churchill Livingstone, Edinburgh 1977).
6   Gross, R.; Gerecke, D.: Tumoren; in Gross, Kaufmann, Löhr, Pathophysiologie, pp. 409–423 (Thieme, Stuttgart 1981).
7   Jansen, J.; Schutt, H.R.E.; Zwet, T.L. van; Mejer, C.J.L.M.; Hijmans, W.: Hairy-cell leukaemia: a B-lymphocytic disorder. Br. J. Haemat. *42:* 21–33 (1979).
8   Leder, L.D.: On the terms 'reticulosis' and 'reticulum cell sarcoma' with regard to the modern concept of the monocyte macrophage system. Klin. Wschr. *56:* 1091–1096 (1978).
9   Long, J.C.: The immunopathology of Hodgkin's disease; in Canellos, Clinics in haematology, vol. 8, pp. 531–566 (Saunders, London 1979).

10    McCulloch, E.A.; Till, J.E.: Stem cells in normal early haemopoiesis and certain clonal haemopathies; in Hoffbrand, Brain, Hirsh, Recent advances in haematology, vol. 2, pp. 85–110 (Churchill Livingstone, Edinburgh 1977).

11    McCulloch, E.A.; Howatson, A.F.; Buick, R.N.; Minden, M.D.; Izaguirre, C.A.: Acute myeloblastic leukemia considered as a clonal hemopathy. Blood Cells 5: 261–282 (1979).

12    Melchner, H. von; Höffken, K.; Schmidt, C.G.: Zur Ätiologie und Pathogenese der Leukämien. Dt. med. Wschr. 44: 1686–1692 (1983).

13    Rappaport, H.: Tumors of the haematopoietic system; in Atlas of tumor pathology, section III, vol. 8 (Armed Forces Institute of Pathology, Washington 1966).

14    Sträuli, P.: Neoplasien; in Siegenthaler, Klinische Pathophysiologie, pp. 1080–1089 (Thieme, Stuttgart 1979).

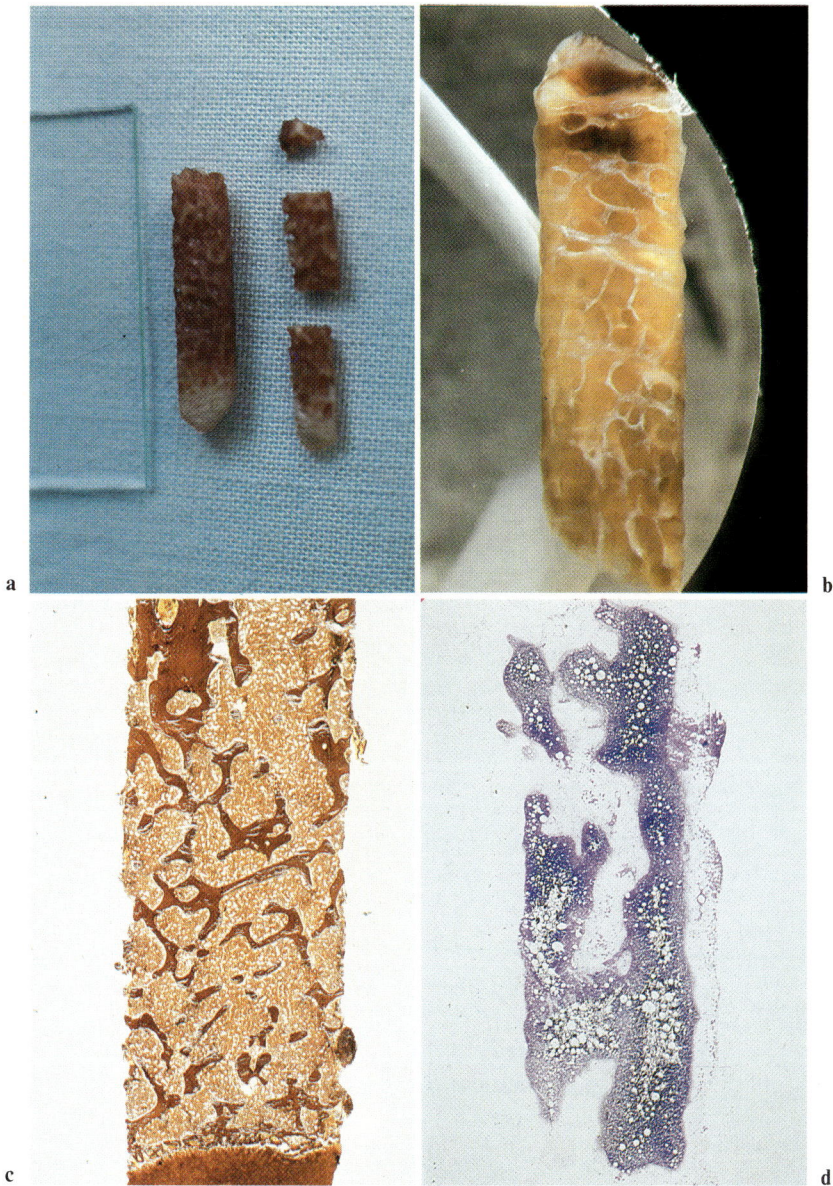

**Plate I.** Processing of the bone marrow biopsy. **a** Longitudinal halving of the biopsy core, the cut surface used for imprints. **b** One biopsy half, embedded in methacrylate. **c** Plastic section of the biopsy. Gomori. $\times 40$. **d** Imprint of the cut surface of one biopsy half. Pappenheim. $\times 10$.

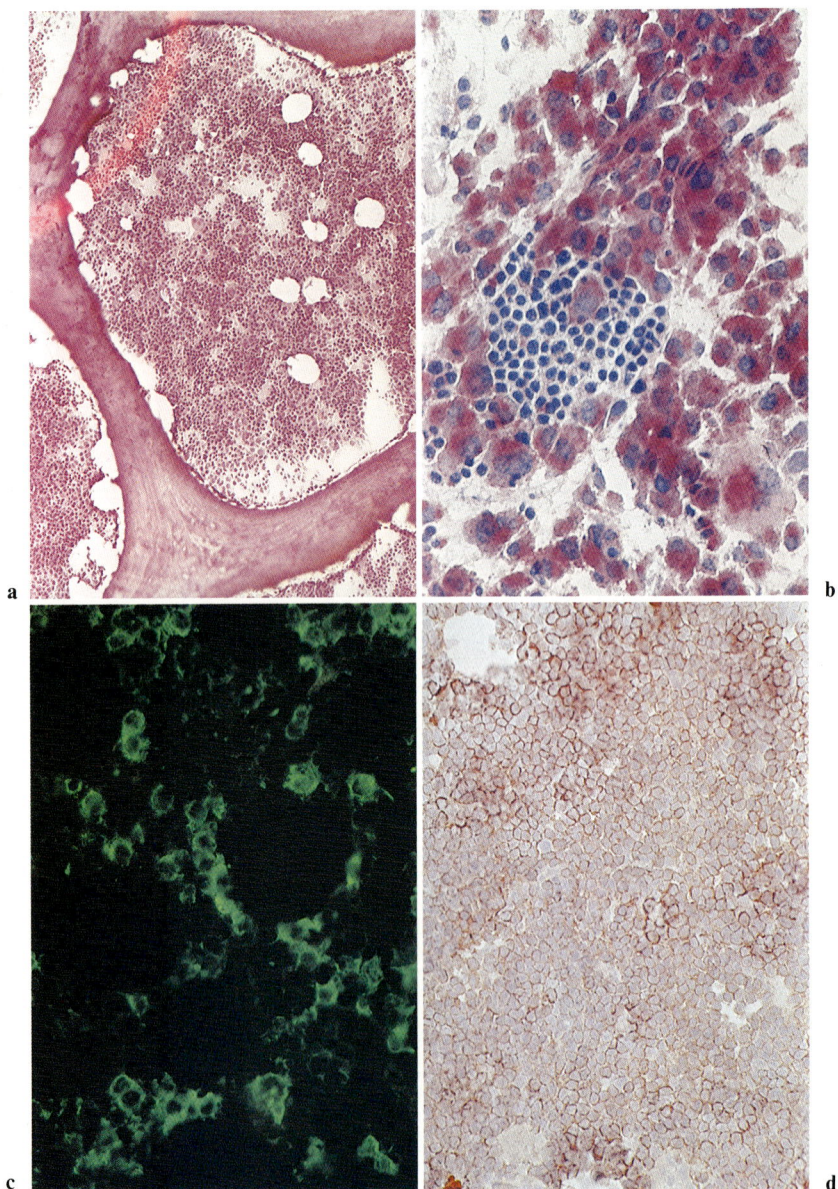

**Plate II.** Histologic investigations on cryostat sections of bone marrow. **a** Fresh frozen section: normal bone and bone marrow. HE. ×100. **b** Histochemistry: multiple myeloma. Acid phosphatase. ×250. **c** Immunohistology: early stage of multiple myeloma, IgA type. Anti-IgA, FITC. ×250. **d** Immunohistochemistry: CLL of B-cell type, kappa type. Anti-kappa, peroxidase. ×250.

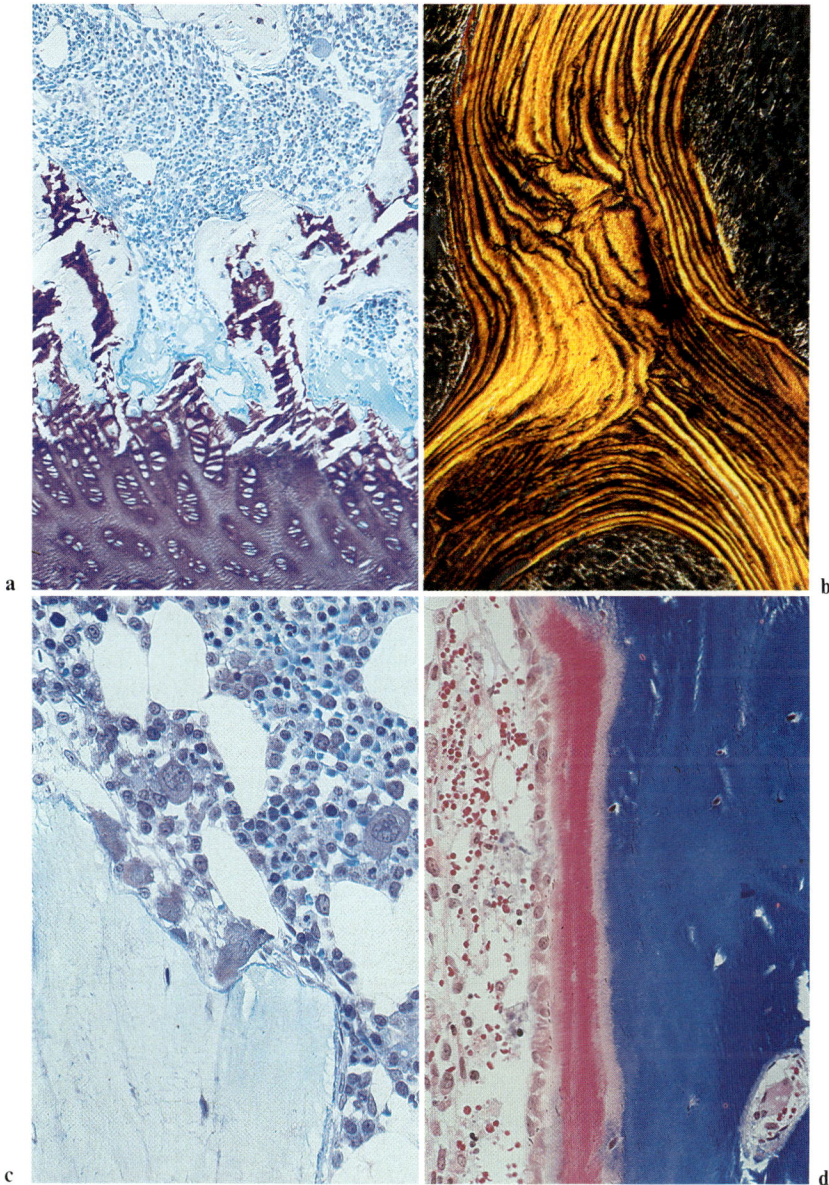

**Plate III.** Normal structure of the trabecular bone. **a** Epiphyseal growth. Giemsa. × 100. **b** Lamellar structure of trabecular bone. Gomori. Polarization. × 250. **c** Osteoclastic bone resorption. Giemsa. × 250. **d** Bone production with broad seam of osteoid (red) and cuboidal osteoblasts; mineralized bone (blue). Ladewig. × 250.

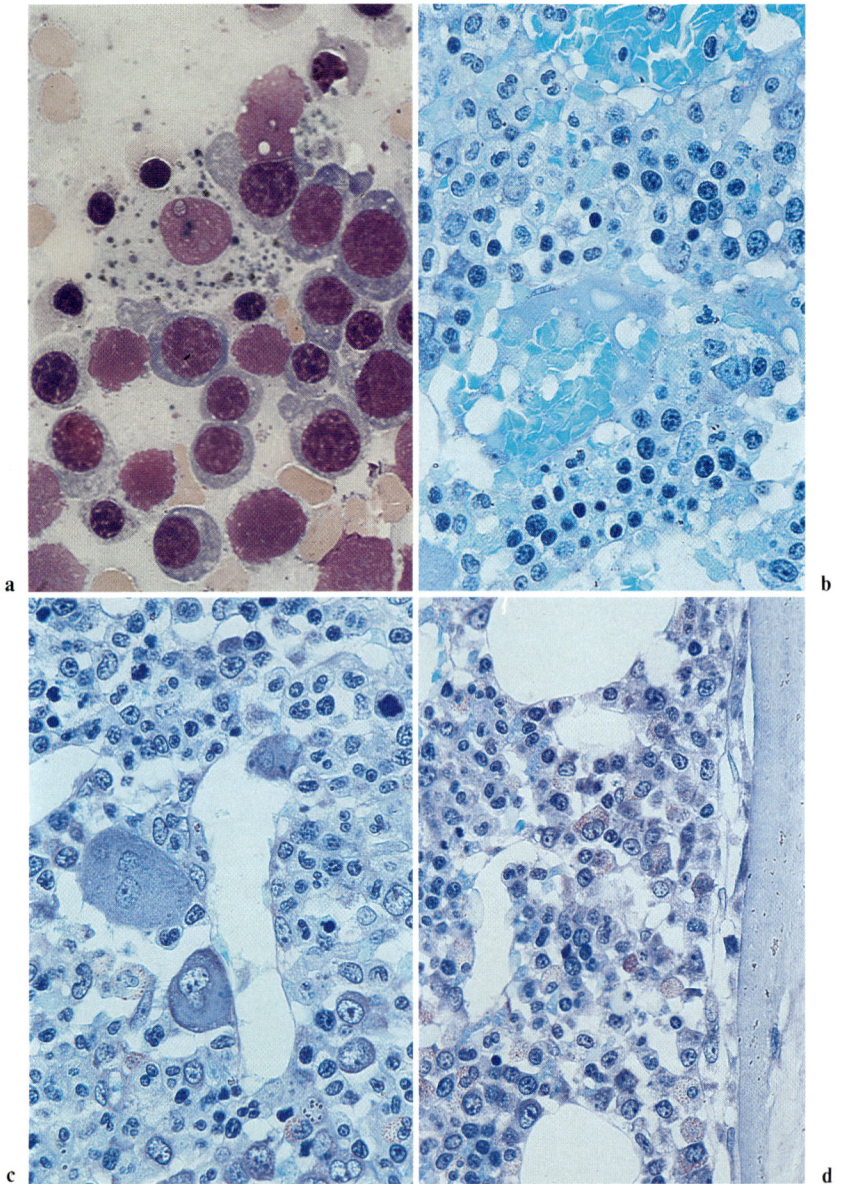

**Plate IV.** Normal structure of the haematopoietic tissue. **a** 'Erythron' with precursors of erythropoiesis and a central histiocyte containing iron. Pappenheim. × 600. **b** 'Erythrons' around a central sinusoid. Giemsa. × 250. **c** Megakaryocytes around a central sinusoid. Giemsa. × 250. **d** Granulopoietic precursors in proximity to a trabecula. Giemsa. × 250.

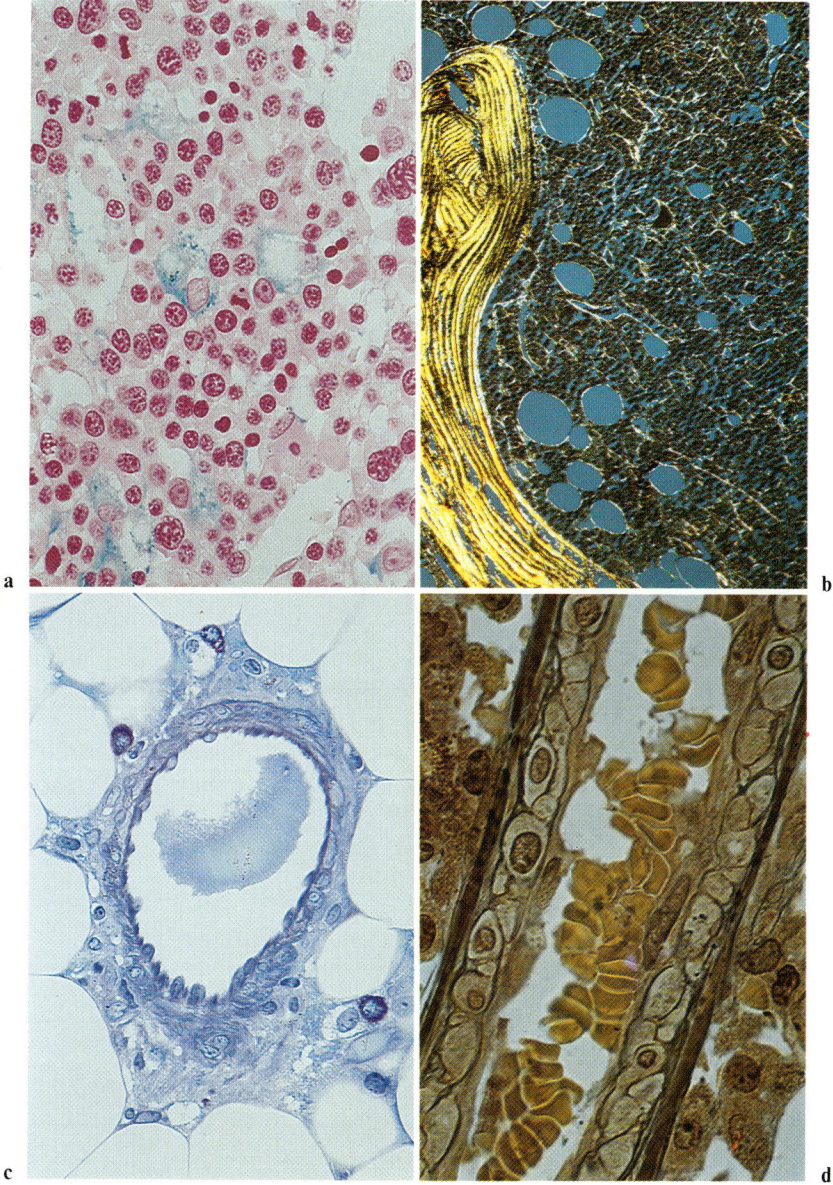

**Plate V.** Normal structure of the bone marrow stroma. **a** Histiocytes containing iron, between erythropoietic precursors. Berlin blue. × 250. **b** Fine network of reticulin fibres. Gomori. Polarization. × 100. **c** Transversely cut artery. Giemsa. × 250. **d** Longitudinally cut artery. Gomori. × 400.

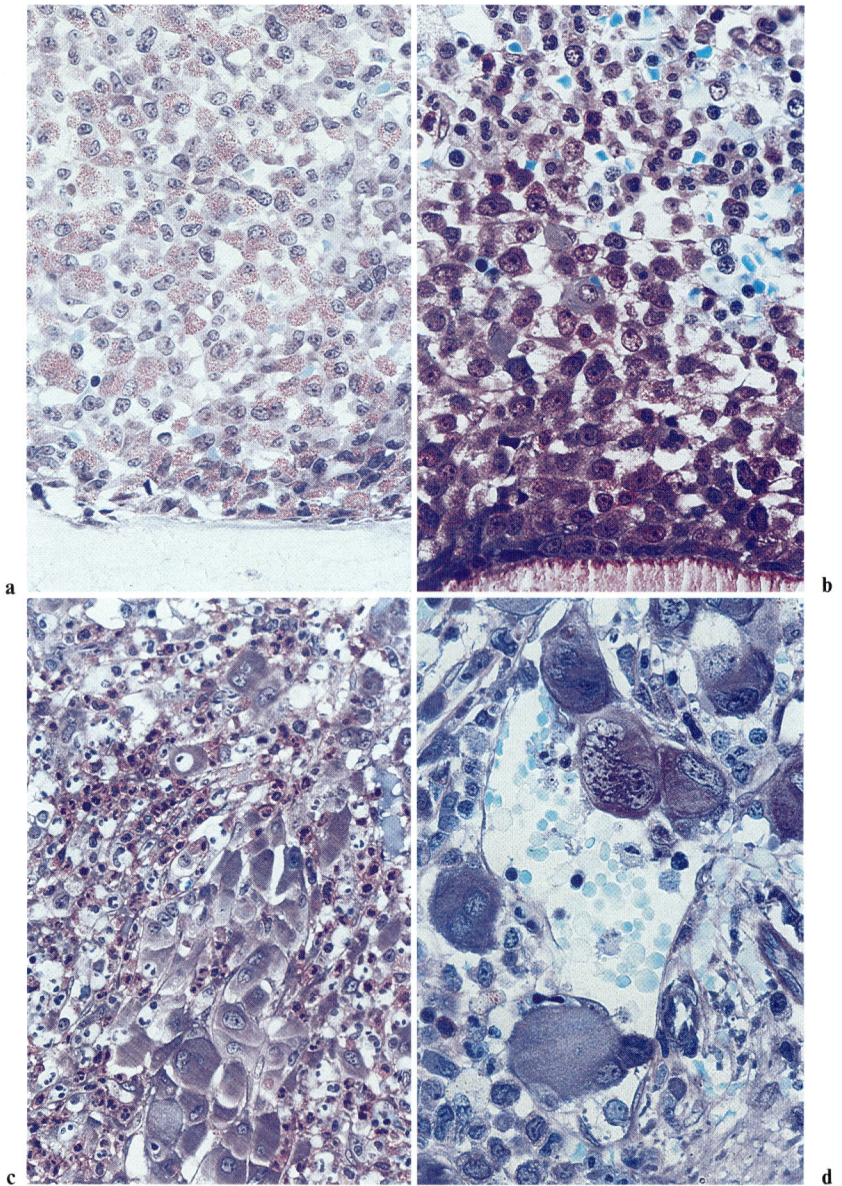

**Plate VI.** Myeloproliferative disorders (MPD). **a** CML, eosinophilic type. Giemsa. ×250. **b** CML, basophilic type. Giemsa. ×250. **c** CML, basophilic/megakaryocytic type. Giemsa. ×100. **d** Proliferation of megakaryocytes in proximity to a central sinusoid. Giemsa. ×250.

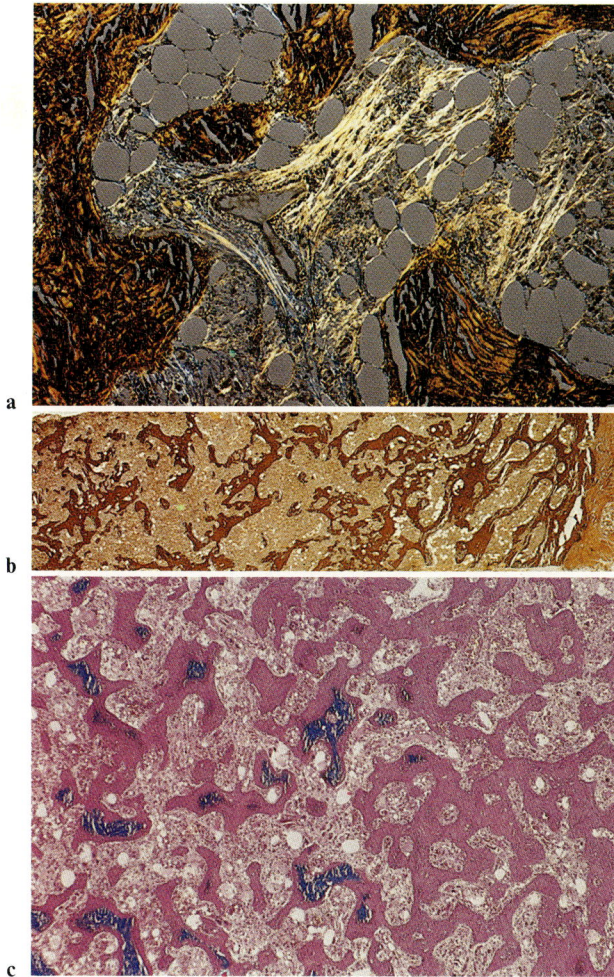

**Plate VII.** Myelofibrosis-osteomyelosclerosis syndrome (MF/OMS). **a** Osteomyelo-sclerosis with coarse fibrosis and primitive bone. Gomori, polarization light. × 250. **b** Irregular architecture of the spongy bone in OMS. Gomori. × 10. **c** Primitive bone in OMS. Red = osteoid, blue = mineralized bone. Ladewig. × 30.

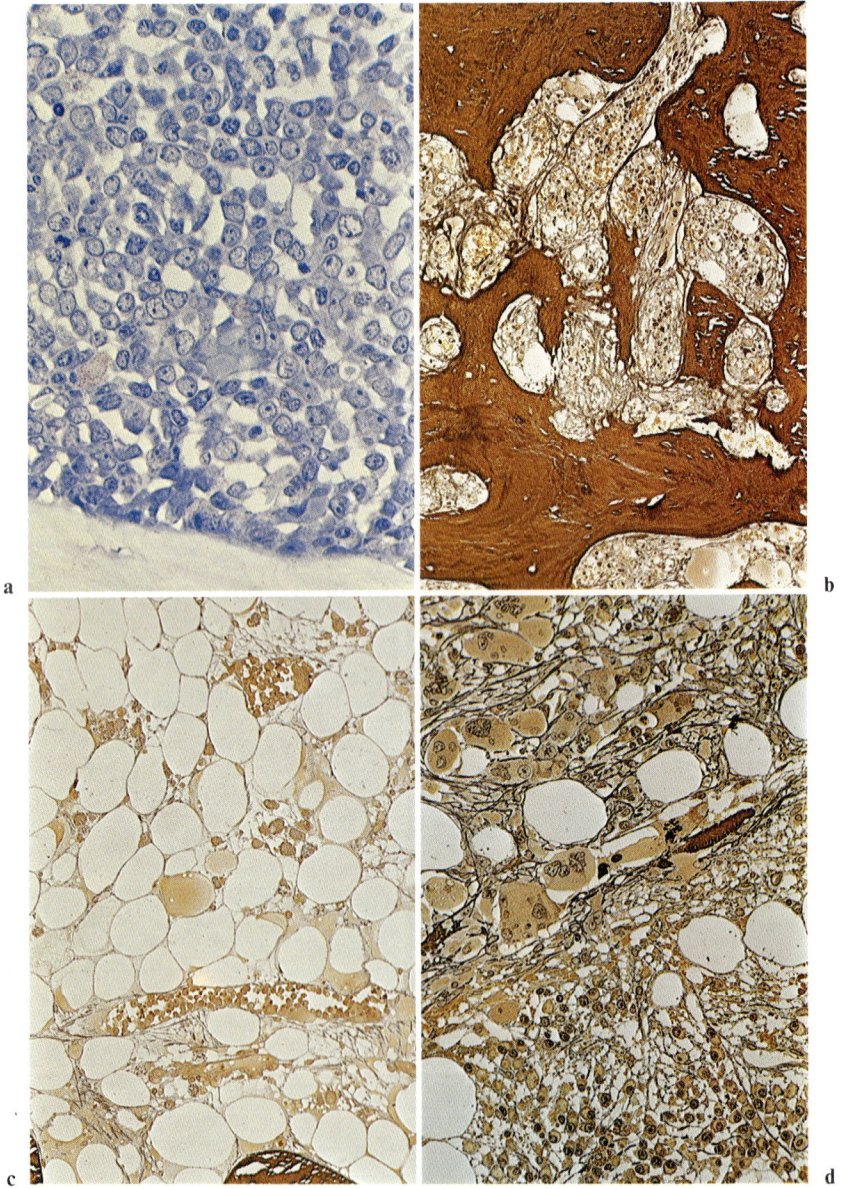

**Plate VIII.** Transitions in chronic myeloproliferative disorders (MPD). **a** To blast crisis in CML. Gallamin blue-Giemsa. × 400. **b** To osteomyelosclerosis in PV. Gomori. × 100. **c** To aplastic crisis in CML, after chemotherapy. Gomori. × 250. **d** To multiple myeloma (below) in MegM. Gomori. × 250.

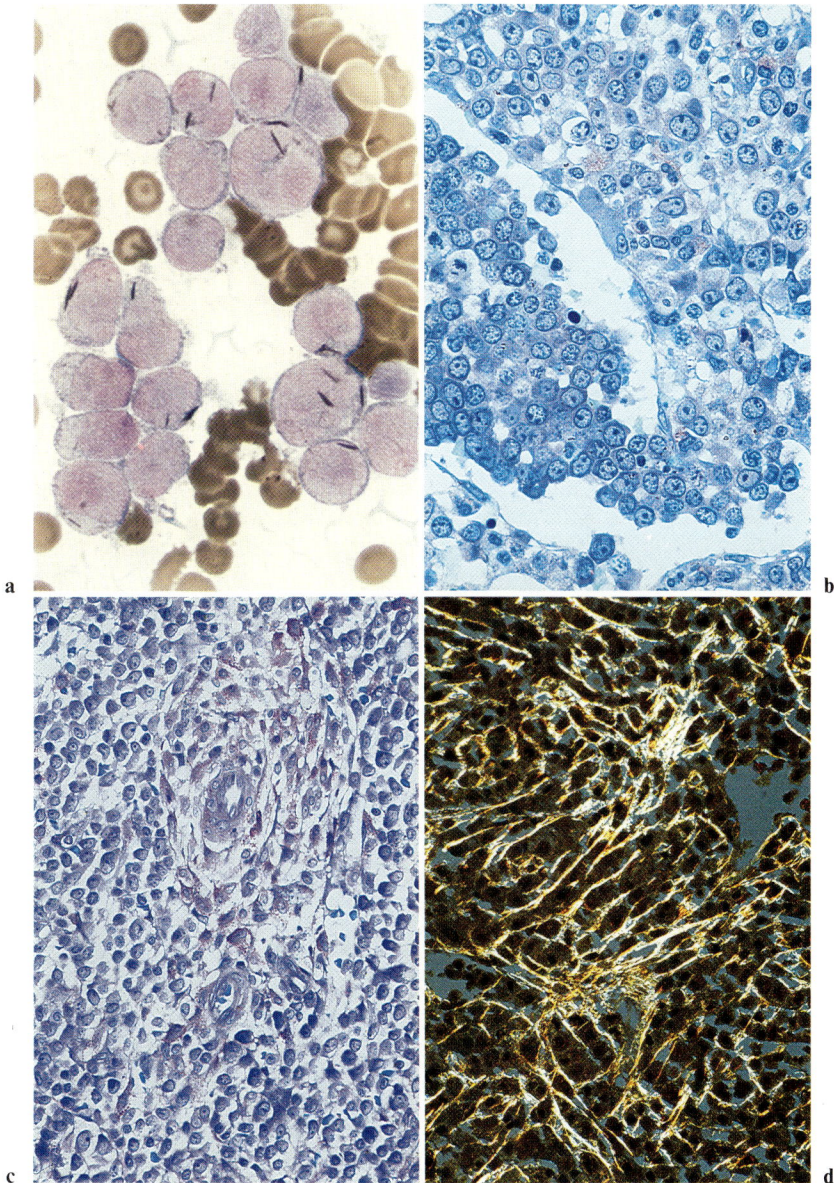

**Plate IX.** Acute leukaemia (AL). **a** Myeloblastic leukaemia with Auer rods. Imprint, Sudan black. × 600. **b** Bilinear acute leukaemia, erythroblastic (in the lumen of the sinusoid), promyelocytic. Giemsa. × 250. **c** Combination of myeloblastic leukaemic and systemic mastocytosis (perivascular). Giemsa. × 100. **d** Marked fibrosis in megakaryoblastic leukaemia ('malignant myelosclerosis'). Gomori. Polarization. × 100.

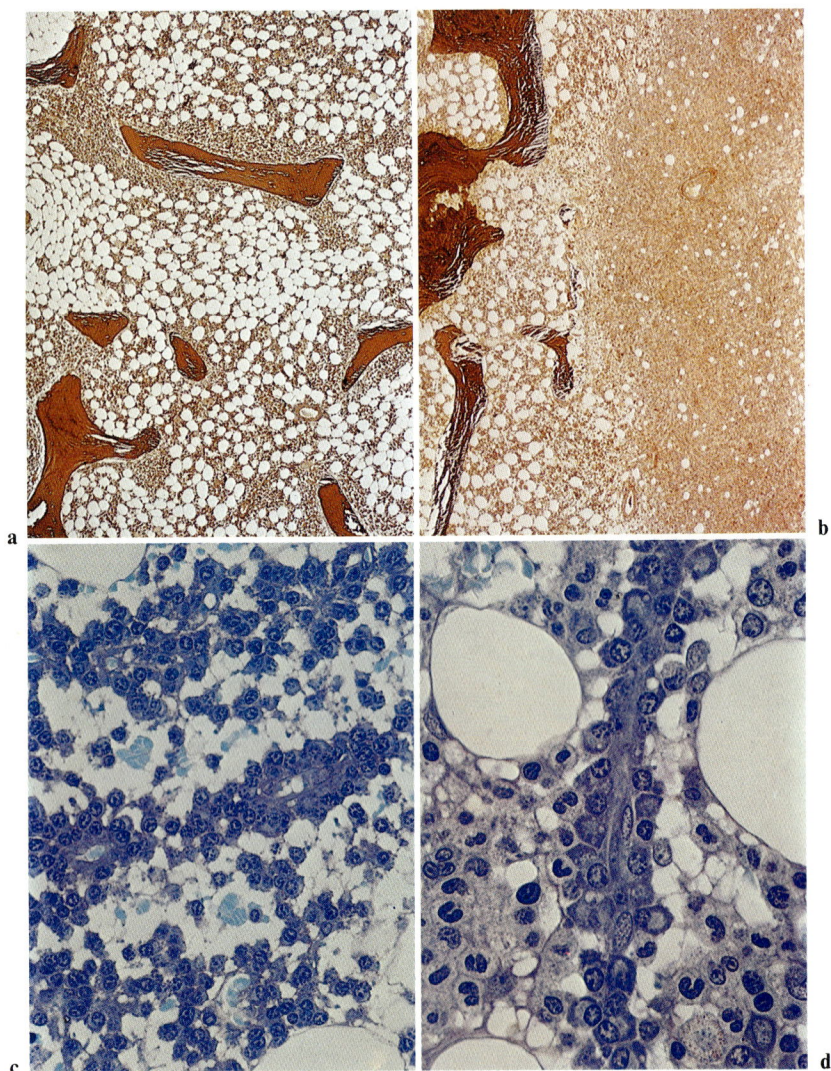

Plate X. Bone marrow histology in multiple myeloma (MM) and in reactive plasma-cytosis (RP). **a** Diffuse proliferation pattern plus dense paratrabecular seams of myeloma cells. Note the striking reduction of haematopoiesis, replacement by fatty tissue (due to hypothetic 'haematopoiesis depressing factor'). Gomori. × 40. **b** Sarcomatous prolifera-tion pattern of plasmablastic sarcoma with marked osteoclastic bone resorption (due to 'osteoclast activating factor'). Gomori. × 40. **c** MM, micro-plasmacytic type, with diffuse proliferation pattern and dense perivascular seams of small, partly lymphocytoid myeloma cells. Gallamin blue-Giemsa. × 400. **d** RP with mature plasma cells, mainly adjacent to a capillary. Gallamin blue-Giemsa. × 400.

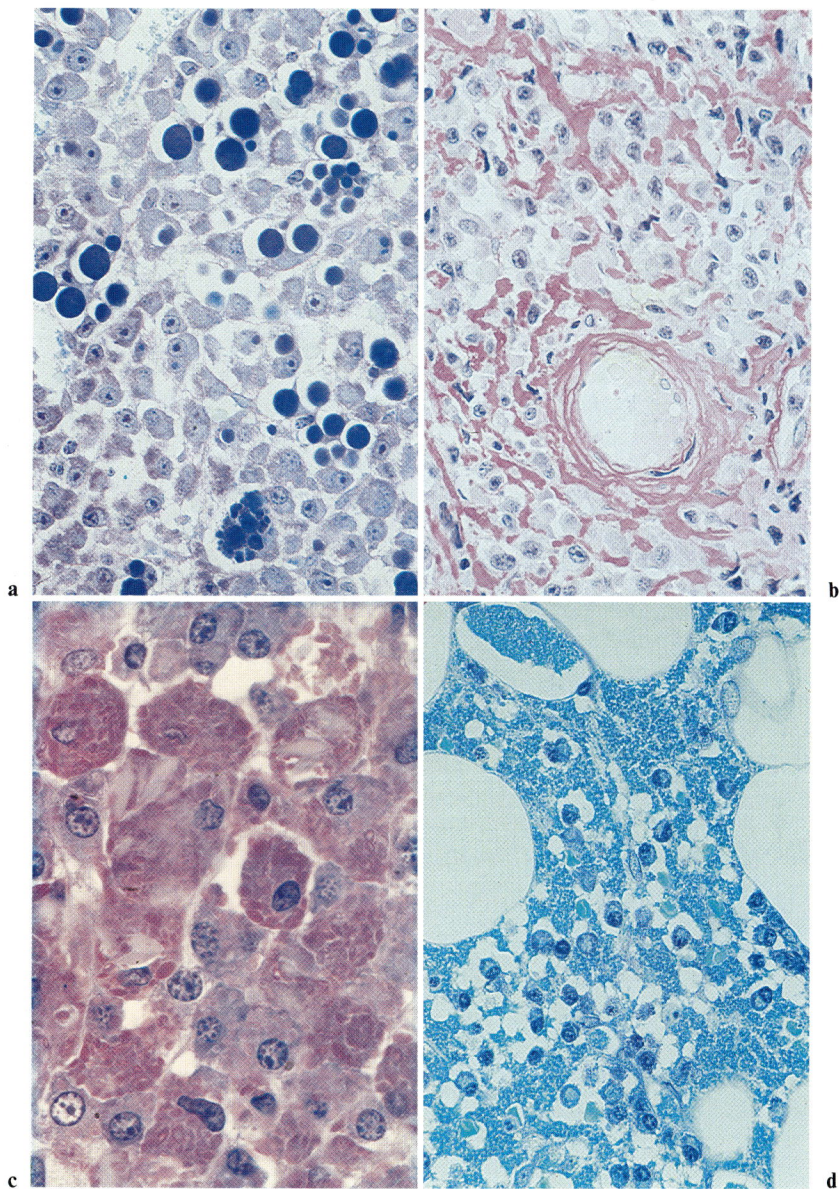

**Plate XI.** Multiple myeloma (MM). **a** Russell bodies in plasmablastic MM. Giemsa. × 400. **b** Interstitial, PAS-positive deposits in MM. PAS. × 250. **c** Intracytoplasmic inclusions in MM. Giemsa. × 600. **d** Intravasal and interstitial deposits of cryoglobulin in MM. Giemsa. × 250.

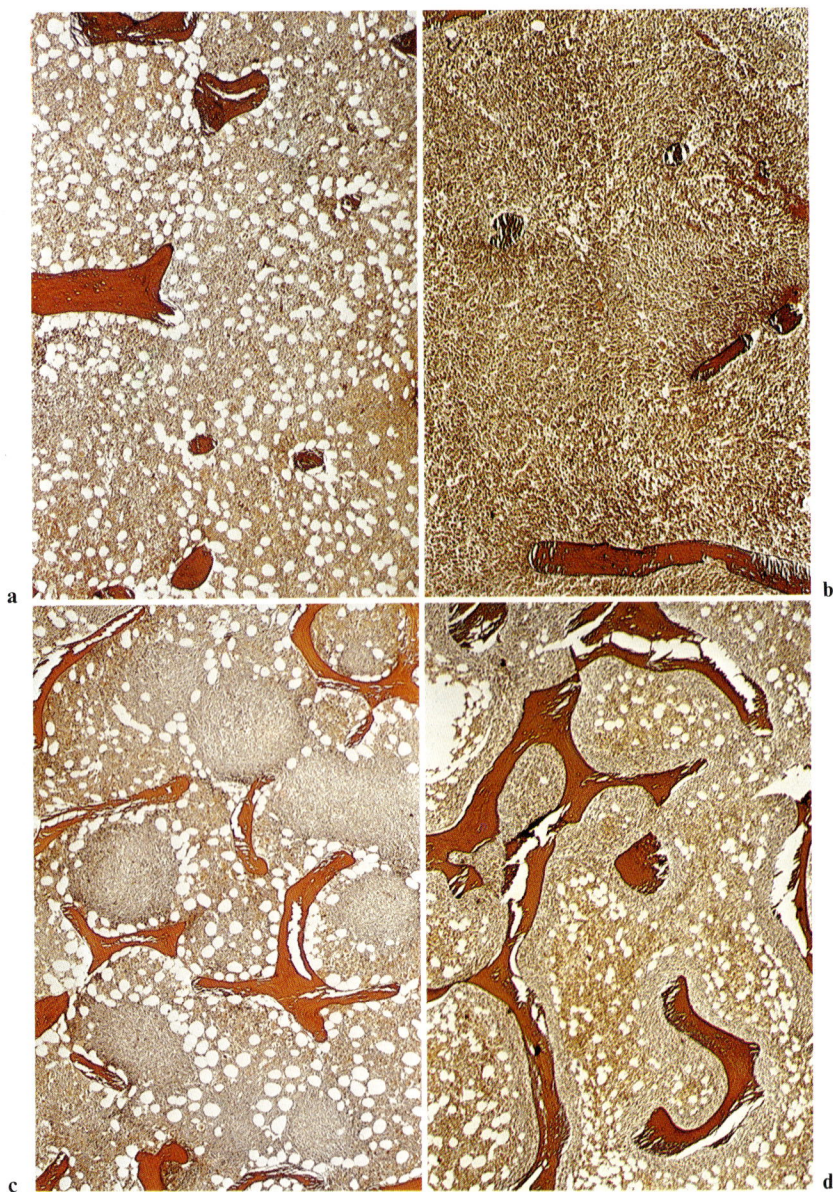

**Plate XII.** Proliferation patterns of non-Hodgkin's lymphomas (NHL) in the bone marrow. Gomori. × 40. **a** Interstitial pattern in ML lymphocytic. **b** Packed marrow pattern in ML lymphocytic. **c** Nodular pattern in ML lymphoplasmacytoid. **d** Paratrabecular pattern in ML centrocytic.

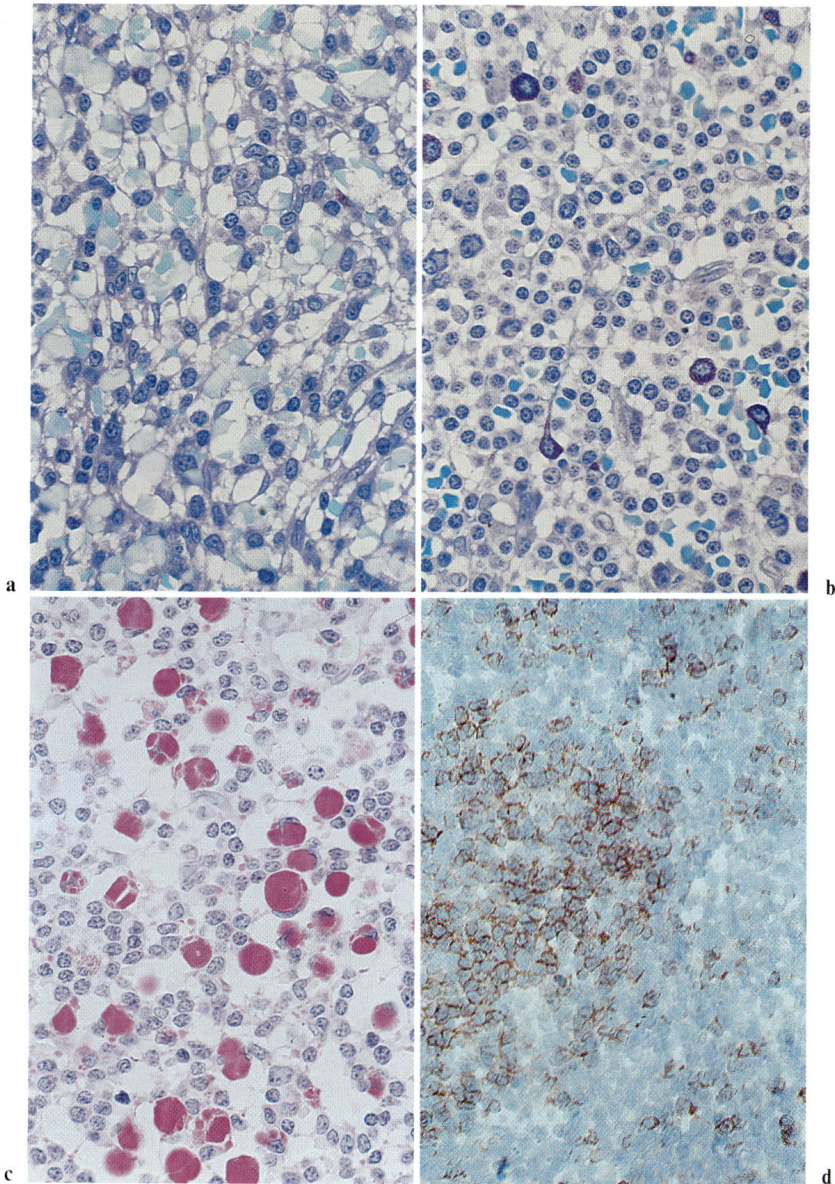

**Plate XIII.** Malignant lymphomas (ML). **a** ML hairy cell. Giemsa. ×250. **b** ML immunocytic. Giemsa. ×250. **c** ML immunocytic with intracytoplasmic inclusions. PAS. ×250. **d** Nodular arrangement of T lymphocytes in ML immunocytic. Frozen section. PAP. Pan-T. ×250.

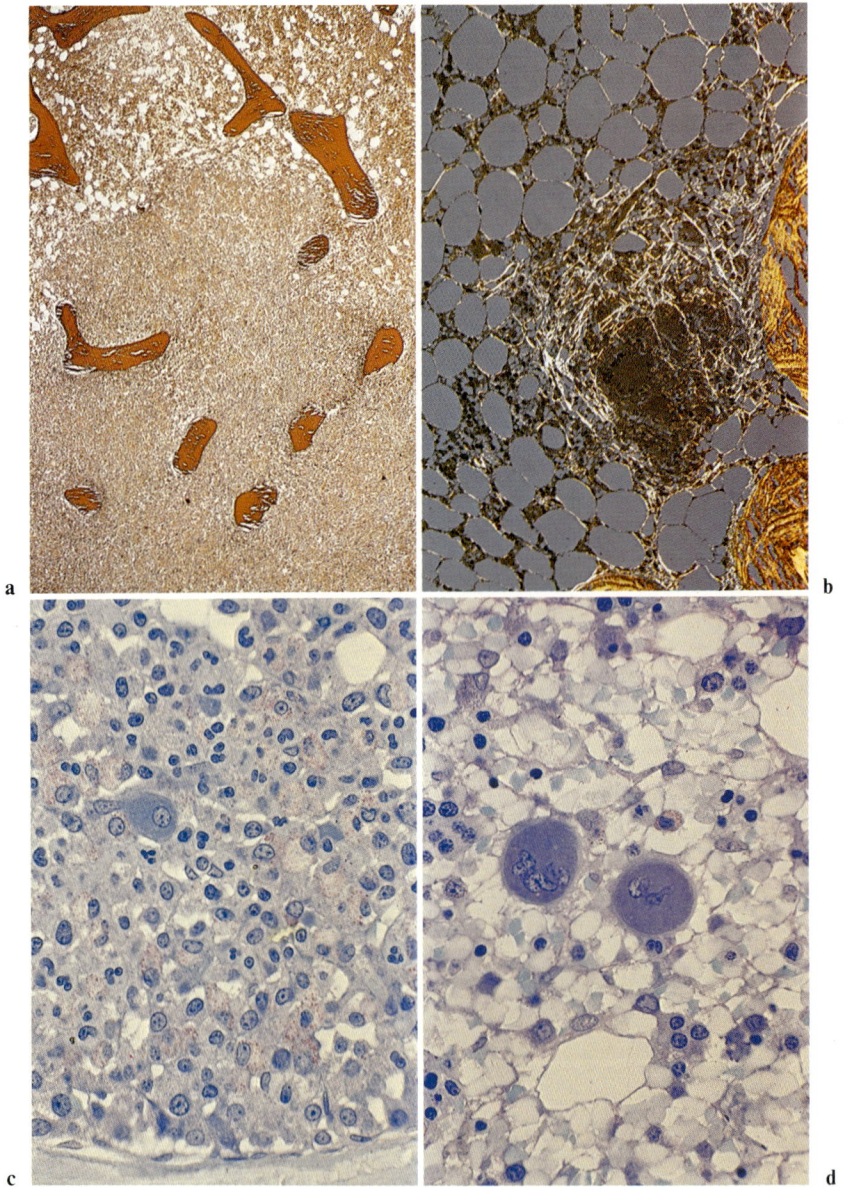

**Plate XIV.** Bone marrow histology in Hodgkin's disease (HD). **a** Large area of bone marrow involvement by HD. Gomori. × 40. **b** Non-caseating epithelioid-cell granuloma. Gomori, polarization light. × 250. **c** Leukaemoid bone marrow reaction in HD. Gallamin blue-Giemsa. × 400. **d** Exsudative bone marrow reaction in HD. Gallamin blue-Giemsa. × 400.

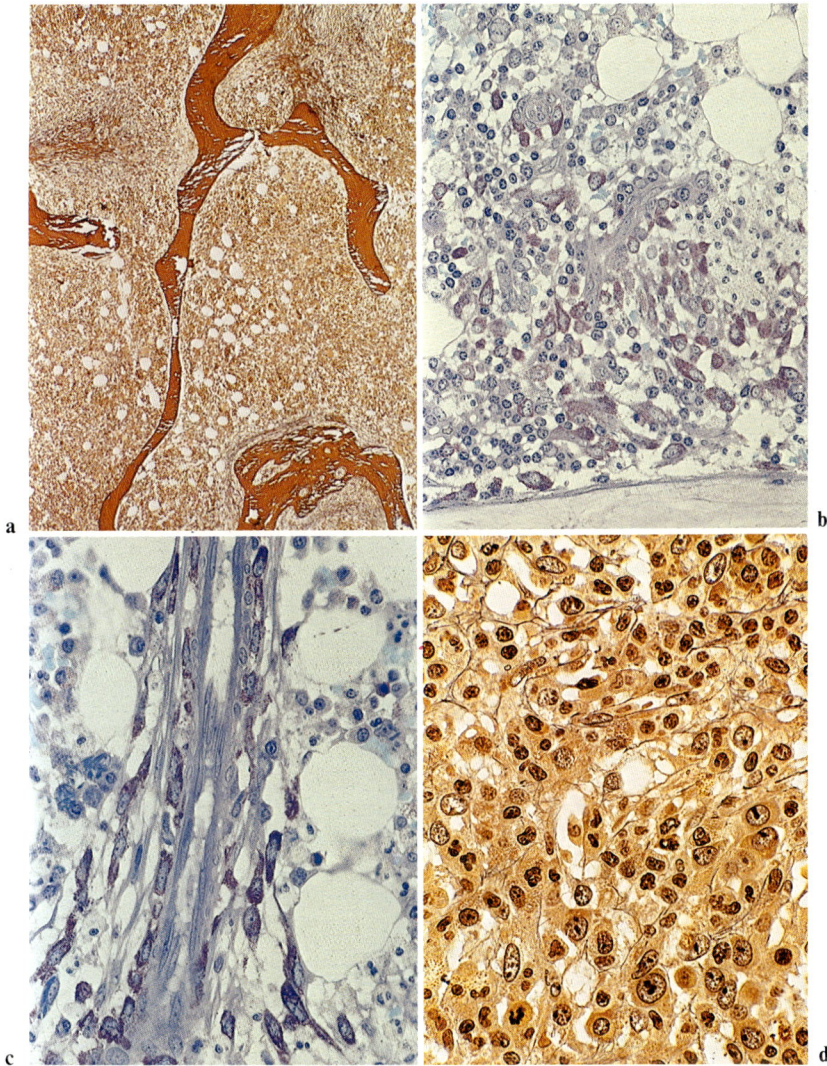

**Plate XV.** Bone marrow lesions in systemic mastocytosis (SM) and in angioimmuno-blastic lymphadenopathy (AILD). **a** Multifocal bone marrow lesions in SM. Note the osteosclerotic reaction to paratrabecular infiltration (below). Gomori. ✕ 40. **b** Mast cell granuloma with spindle-shaped mast cells, lymphocytes and plasma cells. Gallamin blue-Giemsa. ✕ 100. **c** Paravascular mast cell infiltration in SM. Gallamin blue-Giemsa. ✕ 250. **d** Bone marrow manifestation in AILD, consisting of lymphocytes, plasma cells, histio-cytes and immunoblasts, within a network of reticulin fibres and capillaries. Gomori. ✕ 400.

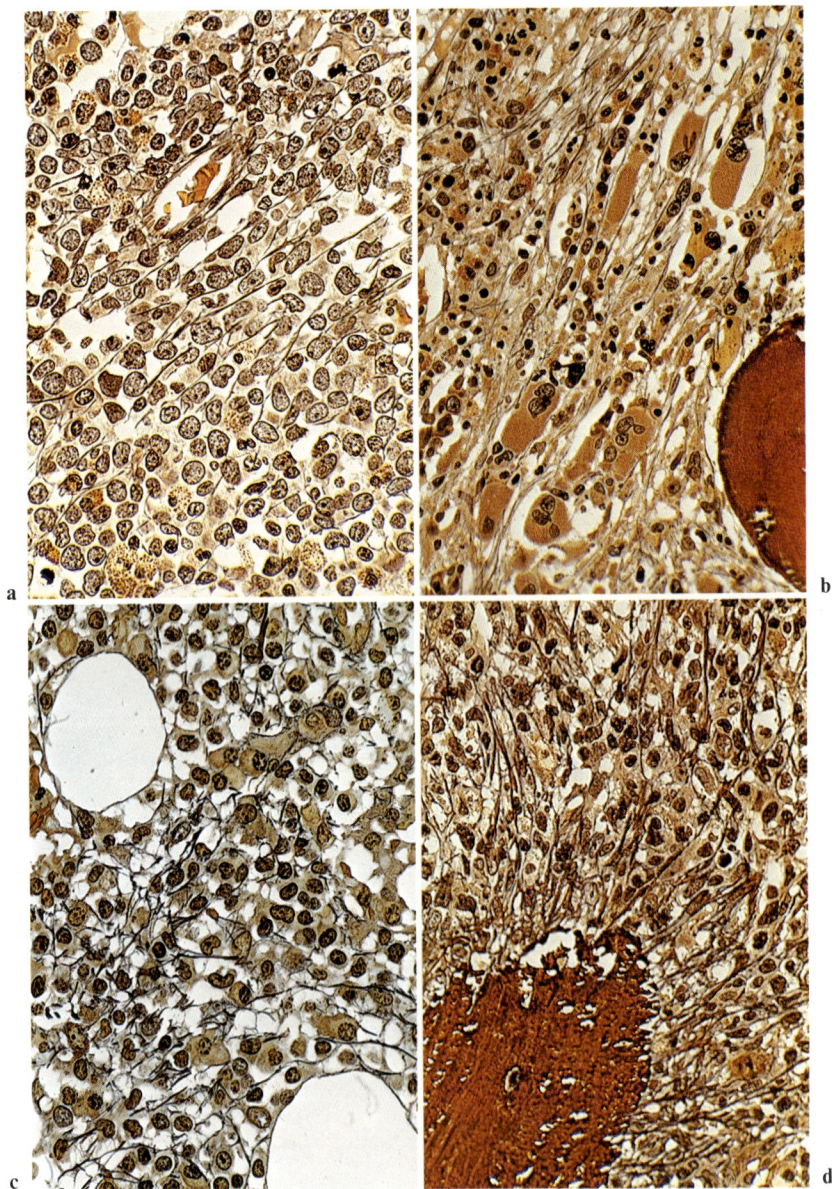

**Plate XVI.** Types of bone marrow fibrosis in haematologic malignancies. Gomori. **a** Fine reticulin fibres in AL myeloblastic. × 250. **b** Coarse fibrosis in MF/OMS. × 200. **c** Close-meshed fibrosis in ML hairy cell. × 250. **d** Dense fibrosis radiating from the trabecular surface in ML centrocytic. × 250.

# Appendix:
# List of Variables Used in Each Patient

| Number | Abbreviation | Description |
|---|---|---|
| 1 | NUM* | number of bone marrow core |
| 2 | AGE* | age (years) |
| 3 | SEX | sex |
| 4 | HBN* | haemoglobin (g/dl) |
| 5 | MCH* | mean cell haemoglobin (pg) |
| 6 | LEU* | leucocytes (1,000/mm$^3$) |
| 7 | THR* | thrombocytes (1,000/mm$^3$) |
| 8 | MYB* | myeloblasts (%, peripheral blood film) |
| 9 | PMC* | promyelocytes (%) |
| 10 | MYC* | myelocytes (%) |
| 11 | MMC* | metamyelocytes (%) |
| 12 | BNE* | band neutrophils (%) |
| 13 | SNE* | segmented neutrophils (%) |
| 14 | EOS* | eosinophils (%) |
| 15 | BAS* | basophils (%) |
| 16 | LYM* | lymphocytes (%) |
| 17 | MON* | monocytes (%) |
| 18 | PBF | pathologic cells in peripheral blood film |
| 19 | RET* | reticulocytes (‰) |
| 20 | SR1* | erythrocyte sedimentation rate (1st hour) |
| 21 | SR2* | erythrocyte sedimentation rate (2nd hour) |
| 22 | FES* | iron, serum (µg/dl) |
| 23 | BIL* | bilirubin, serum (mg/dl) |
| 24 | CRE* | creatinine, serum (mg/dl) |
| 25 | CAL* | calcium, serum (mEq/l) |
| 26 | PHO* | phosphate, serum (mg/dl) |
| 27 | ALK | alkaline phosphatase, serum (IU/l) |
| 28 | TRA | transaminase, serum (IU/l) |
| 29 | LDH | lactate dehydrogenase, serum (IU/l) |
| 30 | TPR* | total proteins, plasma (g/dl) |

* = Unclassified variable.

| Number | Abbreviation | Description |
|--------|--------------|-------------|
| 31 | ALB* | albumin (%) |
| 32 | A1G* | alpha-1-globulin (%) |
| 33 | A2G* | alpha-2-globulin (%) |
| 34 | BEG* | beta-globulin (%) |
| 35 | GAG* | gamma-globulin (%) |
| 36 | IGA* | immunoglobulin A (g/l) |
| 37 | IGG* | immunoglobulin G (g/l) |
| 38 | IGM* | immunoglobulin M (g/l) |
| 39 | PPT | paraprotein-type |
| 40 | LTC | light-chain-type |
| 41 | BJP | Bence-Jones protein |
| 42 | IMP | immunoglobulin peculiarities |
| 43 | MCD | main clinical diagnosis |
| 44 | REL | reliability of clinical diagnosis |
| 45 | CLS | clinical stage |
| 46 | SYM | constitutional symptoms |
| 47 | ACD | additional clinical diagnosis |
| 48 | MFI | major clinical findings |
| 49 | MSY | major symptoms |
| 50 | SYB | duration of symptoms prior to biopsy |
| 51 | SKE | skeletal changes |
| 52 | MSK | method of skeletal investigation |
| 53 | LYN | lymph node changes |
| 54 | MLY | methods of lymph node investigation |
| 55 | SPL | splenic changes |
| 56 | MSP | methods of splenic investigation |
| 57 | HEP | hepatic changes |
| 58 | MHE | method of hepatic investigation |
| 59 | OOR | changes in other organs |
| 60 | MOR | methods in other organs |
| 61 | SMA | sternal marrow aspirate |
| 62 | SHI | special haematologic investigations |
| 63 | CYC | cytochemistry |
| 64 | OHI | histologic organ investigation |
| 65 | OHF | histologic findings |
| 66 | TPB | specific therapy prior to biopsy |
| 67 | SCR | single-agent cytotoxic Rx |
| 68 | MCR | multiple-agent cytotoxic Rx (protocols) |
| 69 | DRB* | duration of Rx before biopsy (months) |
| 70 | STR | steroid Rx |
| 71 | RAD | radiation Rx |

| Number | Abbreviation | Description |
|--------|--------------|-------------|
| 72 | PHR | radio-phosphorus Rx |
| 73 | SPX | splenectomy |
| 74 | SUR | survival to time of study |
| 75 | SUB* | survival from time of biopsy (months) |
| 76 | SUS* | survival from time of first symptom (months) |
| 77 | INT* | interval between first and sequential biopsy (months) |
| 78 | QLT | quality of biopsy core |
| 79 | MHD | main histologic diagnosis |
| 80 | BMI | bone marrow involvement in biopsy |
| 81 | HIS | histologic stage |
| 82 | HST | histologic subtype |
| 83 | CCH | congruence between clinical and histological data |
| 84 | CBV* | cancellous bone (vol%) |
| 85 | HTV* | haematopoietic tissue (vol%) |
| 86 | FTV* | fatty tissue (vol%) |
| 87 | OSV* | osteoid (vol%) |
| 88 | FIV* | fibrotic tissue (vol%) |
| 89 | SIV* | sinusoids (vol%) |
| 90 | EDV* | oedema (vol%) |
| 91 | INV* | neoplastic infiltration (vol%) |
| 92 | WOV* | woven bone (vol%) |
| 93 | OBI* | osteoblastic index (%) |
| 94 | OCI* | osteoblastic index (per 100 mm) |
| 95 | MEN* | megakaryocytes (per $mm^2$ bone marrow) |
| 96 | ERQ | erythropoiesis, quantity |
| 97 | ERM | erythropoiesis, maturity |
| 98 | GRQ | granulopoiesis, quantity |
| 99 | GRM | granulopoiesis, maturity |
| 100 | EOP | eosinophilia |
| 101 | MEQ | megakaryopoiesis, quantity |
| 102 | MEM | megakaryopoiesis, maturity |
| 103 | AME | atypical megakaryocytes |
| 104 | PRP | proliferation pattern |
| 105 | FIN | focal infiltration |
| 106 | HIT | histotopography of neoplastic infiltration |
| 107 | BIN | border of infiltration |
| 108 | DIN | density of infiltration |
| 109 | HIN | homogeneity of infiltration |
| 110 | NEC | necrosis |
| 111 | PAS | PAS positivity |
| 112 | DNC | description of main neoplastic cell type |

| Number | Abbreviation | Description |
|---|---|---|
| 113 | ANC | degree of atypia of main neoplastic cell type |
| 114 | MNC | mitotic activity of neoplastic cells |
| 115 | ANT | description of additional neoplastic cell type |
| 116 | SRI | type of stromal reaction within infiltrates |
| 117 | DSR | degree of stromal reaction within infiltrates |
| 118 | SFI | structure of fibrosis within infiltrates |
| 119 | FCI | presence of fat cells within infiltrates |
| 120 | VIN | structure of vessels within infiltrates |
| 121 | GRT | description of granulomatous tissue |
| 122 | SBO | description of spongy bone |
| 123 | OSR | description of osseous remodelling |
| 124 | SRB | stromal reaction at borders of infiltrates |
| 125 | AVQ | arterial vessels in the bone marrow, quantity |
| 126 | AVC | arterial vessels in the bone marrow, changes |
| 127 | SIQ | sinusoids, quantity |
| 128 | SIC | sinusoids, changes |
| 129 | PLA | plasma cells, quantity and distribution |
| 130 | MAS | mast cells, quantity and distribution |
| 131 | PHA | phagocytic cells |
| 132 | MAT | degree of marrow atrophy |
| 133 | LYN* | lymphoid nodules |

# Subject Index